"After reading Dr. Bob's advice on surgery, I felt empowered to make the experience the best it could be for me and my family. Thanks, Dr. Bob, for directing us through the health-care maze."
Kathy Aymard, R.N.

"*The Medical Mentor* is a clear, informed, and absolutely essential guide for those whose health depends on their ability to negotiate our Byzantine medical-care system."
Gordon Livingston, M.D.

"This book is hard to put down. Dr. Bob's inviting, conversational style takes readers inside the system, clarifying issues that are vital to health care. Anyone who envisions needing medical intervention should have a copy of *The Medical Mentor* on his bookshelf."
Lou Aymard, Ph.D.

"I was very fortunate to have Bob Sheff's supportive guidance during the stressful time, several years ago, when I was deciding on the best way to deal with the diagnosis of prostate cancer. This book grows out of Dr. Bob's years of work as a highly respected clinician who is able and glad to offer his knowledge, compassion, and practical wisdom to others, like me, when confronted with a complicated and frightening decision."
Herb Horowitz, Ph.D.

"My family and I, and many others I know, have benefited greatly from Bob's practical, professional, and compassionate assistance in navigating today's complicated and often-impersonal health-care system. He has helped us obtain not only the care we need when we need it but also greater peace of mind."
The Honorable Elizabeth Bobo
Maryland House of Delegates

"Bob Sheff leads you to the heart of the matter—the patient's needs. He taught me when to question, whom to ask, how to ask it. Then he taught me the most important thing—to listen to my husband and to accept his decisions without regret."
Lin Eagan
Maryland Realtor

The Medical Mentor

Get the Health Care You Deserve in Today's Medical System

Bob Sheff, M.D.

The Medical Mentor

Get the Health Care You Deserve in Today's Medical System

Bob Sheff, M.D.

STC Healthy Living
STEWART, TABORI & CHANG
NEW YORK

Editor: Debora Yost
Designers: Larissa Nowicki and Carl Williamson
Production Manager: Jane Searle

Published in 2006 by
Stewart, Tabori & Chang, an Imprint of Harry N. Abrams

Library of Congress Cataloging-in-Publication Data
Sheff, Bob.
    The medical mentor: get the health care you deserve in today's medical
system / by Bob Sheff
      p. cm
    Includes index.
    ISBN: 1–58479–488–7
    1. Medical personnel and patient   2. Medical care—Popular works.
    3. Consumer education. I. Title: Get the health care you deserve in today's
medical system. II. Title.

R727.S54 2006
610.69'6—dc22
                                                    2005034434

The text of this book was composed in Meta.

Printed in the United States

10 9 8 7 6 5 4 3 2 1

First Printing

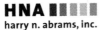
HNA
harry n. abrams, inc.
a subsidiary of La Martinière Groupe

115 West 18th Street
New York, NY 10011
www.abramsbooks.com

For my wife, Arlene, who brings out the best in me

Acknowledgments

First and foremost, I want to acknowledge the family, friends, and patients who shared their stories with me and trusted me to be their medical advocate. Special thanks to my wife, Arlene, whose knowledge and wisdom as a psychotherapist and partnership in my work with patients led to the creation of this book. I also want to thank my literary agent, John Monteleone, for understanding the message we wanted to share and for his faith and persistence in finding this work a home. Many thanks to Debora Yost, my editor at Stewart, Tabori & Chang. Without her support and guidance, this book would never have achieved its final form. And, finally, to my children and grandchildren, who make this work and life worth doing.

CONTENTS

FOREWORD
Why You Need This Book

My mother died unexpectedly and alone in a Chicago hospital at age 61. She had been admitted for tests, and it was never made clear to me what exactly happened to cause her death. This was before I knew Dr. Bob Sheff and before I had the privilege of serving in the Maryland legislature and working primarily on health issues. If I had known then what I know now about the medical system in America, I would have handled my mother's hospitalization differently. I did not understand how important it is to be prepared to be your own health advocate, and your family's.

I now know, as you probably do, that our health-care system is in disarray, and it is not patient-friendly. My position as a legislator has given me a broader perspective on this problem. My involvement in health issues during my early committee assignments in the Maryland General Assembly led me to a growing relationship with Dr. Sheff. As I delved deeper into laws and regulations affecting health care and health insurance, it became apparent that the issues I was working to resolve were symptoms of a larger and more complex problem. I often turned to Dr. Sheff to guide me through the complicated web of health insurance and health care, just as you are turning to his book to guide you.

Though I knew him first as the Medical Director of our community medical group, Dr. Sheff quickly became an invaluable professional resource, voicing concerns and providing insight from his own multi-faceted experiences as a physician, a health-care administrator, and, unavoidably later, as a patient. Together we understand nearly every point of view—the doctor's, the patient's and the insurance company's—and, as we worked together we tried to study situations from these multiple perspectives. It became apparent that no matter whose place you take or what situation you are in, there is but one basic truth: The health-care system in the United States is not working as it should.

To me and to many others involved in trying to correct this problem, the patient's welfare is paramount. Doctors want to achieve positive outcomes for the people who trust and rely on them. Hospital administrators want high success rates for procedures performed under their jurisdiction, and they work hard to maintain a high standard of care. Even the insurance companies, so often seen as the enemy, have to worry about more than just the bottom line, because customer satisfaction is a part of doing business.

The problem isn't the people who work in the system. It's the system itself. No isolated legislation will solve this problem; it requires sweeping reforms that simply aren't forthcoming, despite concerted effort by legislators, lobbyists, and citizens. Unfortunately, this will not be resolved anytime soon.

What, then, are you, the patient, to do? You need to take the health care of you and your loves ones into your own hands; you need to be your own medical advocate. You need the knowledge and skills to navigate the confusing system of doctors, referrals, hospitals, and health-insurance policies, forms, and regulations that will get you the outcome you want and deserve. And when you can't do it alone, or you are too sick to be your own advocate, you need friends and loved ones with this same knowledge to represent you.

It is best to learn these skills now, rather than in the midst of a crisis. Being hurt or ill, or watching a loved one in pain, is hard enough without having to battle the health-care system blindfolded for the care that is needed. *The Medical Mentor* is your best teacher. I know this from personal experience.

When my daughter, Cayley, was in college, she spent a semester studying abroad in Hungary. While there, she became very ill. Her symptoms were severe enough that she needed urgent care. She was initially turned away from the Hungarian health services because she was a noncitizen. Cayley was finally able to find a Hungarian doctor, whose management of the problem only made things worse. She then found the American Clinic in Budapest, and was evaluated there.

As any mother would, I wanted to make sure that she was receiving the best care and getting all the medical attention she needed. For her to be sick, alone, and far away was frightening for both of us. I felt doubly ill-equipped to help her because I speak neither Hungarian nor medicalese. After treatment began at the American Clinic, Cayley and I still had concerns about whether she was receiving the appropriate care. She was in too much pain to think for herself and she needed an advocate.

I turned to Dr. Sheff for help. Dr. Sheff went above and

beyond and phoned Cayley's doctor in Hungary (despite a 6-hour time difference) to discuss her care and the plan of action. I learned from Dr. Sheff's example how the medical advocate needs to be assertive in insisting that doctors communicate their understanding of the medical problem, the diagnosis, the treatment plan, and their expectation.

As it turned out, the course of treatment the doctor at the American Clinic implemented was the right thing to do. Knowing that she had a medical advocate working on her behalf built Cayley's confidence in her treatment and my reassurance that she was in good hands. It also helped ease the strain of this stressful time and, I'm sure, helped her heal.

It turns out that I am only one of many people who knows Dr. Sheff and have turned to him for help during times of medical crises. Now that his helpful advice is in a book, he can help everyone. In our current, flawed health-care system, the stakes are high, and your odds on having a good outcome are best if you know how to be your own advocate. *The Medical Mentor* is the best tool that exists to make that happen.

The Honorable Shane Pendergrass

Maryland House of Delegates

Member, Health Care Delivery and Financing

Joint Committee Member, Health and Government Operations Committee

Chairwoman, Health Insurance Subcommittee

1

WHY YOU NEED
A MEDICAL MENTOR

Will the health-care system get better soon?

What should I do?

Do I really need to know this now?

What if these approaches don't work?

Can I do this without your help?

The American Medical-Care System Is a Mess!

Illness is scary enough without adding to it the confusing way the current medical system works. If you're feeling as though it is getting harder and harder to obtain the health care you want and need, I can assure that you are not alone.

All of us have experienced exasperating hours waiting to see the doctor, feeling rushed while with the doctor, then walking out with unanswered questions. You may have experienced procedures being done and talked about as if you were not even there, and being ordered to take pills without getting an explanation as to why.

It's no wonder we feel helpless. And it happens during the times when we need help the most!

It's understandable why we sometimes feel unprepared to make wise decisions about our medical care; we don't realize that we're even entitled to do so. This is only compounded by the difficulties we often experience when our insurance companies reject paying for medical care and procedures we thought we were entitled to. And so we end up, one little person left to fight a faceless, all-powerful behemoth insurance company. And we have to do so when we are at our most vulnerable, either ill ourselves or worried about someone who is.

- **Will the health-care system get better soon?**
  The answer is, to the best of my judgment, no! Certainly it does not appear that the U.S. government has the political will, or even the capability, to improve the medical-care system and make it friendly and accessible to all patients. The insurance companies (including private insurers and local, state, and federal health programs), by creating so many barriers to accessing care, seem to be part of the problem, not the solution. And doctors, depending on your point of view, are either part of the problem or are as unhappy about the current state of health care as patients. Nevertheless, they seem to be powerless to correct the problem.

- **What should I do?**

  The answer to this question is what *The Medical Mentor* is all about. If the system is a mess (and it is), and if there does not appear to be a solution in the near future (and there does not), then **you must learn how to be your own successful medical advocate.** If you have the right knowledge and skills, you can get the health care you want—not the care that someone else wants to give you or says that you need. *The Medical Mentor* will teach you the skills so you can get:

  - An appointment with the doctor you want.
  - Your doctors to communicate effectively with you.
  - Your medical care managed properly in the various setting in which you care to receive it.
  - Your insurance company to pay its share.

  That's just the beginning. *The Medical Mentor* will give you the skills to work your way through the whole maze of the medical-care system so that you will never feel lost again.

  > The medical-care system is a mess and it's unlikely a positive change will happen anytime soon! You must learn to take charge of your own health.

- **Do I really need to know this now?**

  In terms of your best interests, yes! One of the hard truths of life is that illness is something we must deal with from time to time. Perhaps you or someone you love is even dealing with an illness now. If this is the case, you should know that it is common for the patient, family, and friends to feel scared, frustrated, confused, and alone at times throughout the ordeal. I have been there, as have many others. *The Medical Mentor* is intended to help make your experience as painless as possible.

What This Book Will Teach You

This book offers all the skills you need to successfully be your own medical advocate. You will find out, through specific instructions and examples, that there is a global strategy to successfully navigate the medical system. You can steer your own course, and I am going to show you how. The anchor of this strategy is **creating critical partnerships with your doctors**. This may not be your past or current experience but, trust me, it can happen, and it will work. Like all partnerships, it only works if all parties understand and agree on the ground rules. I will teach you the ground rules and how to implement them. I will also teach you what to do if the partnership is not working.

> *The Medical Mentor* will teach you the strategies to become your own successful patient advocate in any health-care situation.

This book is about getting the best medical care, but it is not about how to get care for a specific health condition. There are a number of disease-specific books on the market that offer technical information on procedures, diagnoses, and treatment options. Rather, this book will teach you how to empower yourself so that you can become totally informed about your disease, know and understand your medical options, and make an informed decision along with your doctor or doctors. Learning the approach that will allow you to better succeed at getting the care you want and need is critical to all patients no matter what their medical condition.

Self-empowerment is what being your own medical advocate is all about. Many patients do not feel that they have the right to ask challenging questions or to request specific care from their health-care providers. The approach you will learn is intended to teach you how to **give yourself permission** to do just that.

This is not a call to battle. It is a guide to working within the system to get the most out of it. Along the way, we will look at many examples of the typical and some not-so-typical problems patients face. We will explore options to solve these problems.

> A combination of knowledge
> and approach will empower you
> to speak up to doctors and
> insurance companies.

- **What if these approaches don't work?**

  There may be times when creating a relationship with your
  medical team does not go the way it should. I will teach you
  how to be *cooperatively assertive*. There may come a time
  when being cooperatively assertive just doesn't seem to work,
  either. Where appropriate, I offer more aggressive, strong-arm
  techniques. It saddens me to do so, but I have increasingly
  encountered situations in which, because I am a physician,
  I can get the attention and changes needed in the care of a
  patient, but the patient and/or his support team cannot. At
  times like these, you will have to get more aggressive until
  someone responds to you. You'll learn what to do when you
  encounter these roadblocks.

> Sometimes you have to increase
> the aggressiveness of your
> approach until you get the right
> person to respond. I will teach you
> the best approach.

- **Can I do this without your help?**

  Unfortunately, that is unlikely. It has been my repeated
  experience that patients and families under the stress of a
  threatened or actual illness find it extremely difficult to make the
  necessary decisions and manage the many demanding
  relationships required in modern medicine without professional
  guidance. No matter how smart you are or how well you
  manage life in other situations, you can get lost navigating the
  complexities of today's medical system. It's a big sea, and the
  barriers in our medical system can fog even the sharpest minds.

  As I have seen over and over again, what seems like common
  sense or clearly understandable in the calm of your usual
  healthy life becomes difficult or impossible to sort out in the
  chaos of a medical crisis. As Rudyard Kipling once said, *"If you
  can keep your wits about you while all others are losing theirs...*

The world will be yours..." In this case, you don't want the entire world, you just want control of your own medical destiny!

A MATTER OF GENDER. To avoid offending either sex and also avoid making reading cumbersome, I alternate gender from chapter to chapter when I am referring to doctors and patients. The only exceptions to this are when I am speaking about my own care or telling real-life stories (though names have been changed to protect their privacy). Hopefully this rotation will make the reading much easier for you.

It Is Not Always Easy...But It Works

A PERSONAL EXPERIENCE...

A few years ago, my family went through the difficult experience of the terminal illness and death of my wife's 86-year-old mother. During her hospitalization, we were confronted with several situations that to us didn't seem to be going as they should. Deciding how to intervene was stressful because it can be difficult, even for a doctor, to confront a medical staff and ask for changes in the way they provide care. We found some of the nurses were very open to our concerns and suggestions, but others were hostile.

For instance, being turned in bed was very painful and frightening to my mother-in-law. Even simple procedures like having her blood pressure and pulse monitored upset her. As her advocates, we asked the medical team in charge to limit these activities. We had discussed with her physician whether these activities were even necessary. Her physician agreed that they were not, and that the goal was to limit her suffering. Even so, we had to be very firm with some of the staff.

I believe they were all good people, but they had established routines, and we were asking them to change their behavior. My wife and I, on several occasions, had to remind ourselves to use the strategies that would get the care her mother deserved. There were occasions when we didn't manage an encounter with the staff as well as we could have. So, we'd go back to the staff and review the issue again with a better plan to achieve the care we wanted.

We learned two things from this experience. First, **it is in your best interest to think about how to manage a health-care situation before you have to deal with it.** Second, during the heat of any moment, even with advance planning, you may sometimes find it very difficult to remember and follow your own plan. When it appears things are not working, you need to pause, review your approach, and then use different techniques to get the result desired.

This book will teach you in advance how to deal with the medical system as illnesses are occurring and changing. It will also teach you how to review and evaluate decisions and, when necessary, reconsider and come up with a better approach.

How I Can Help You

I have spent my professional career in the health-care industry. I started out as a physician. I went to medical school at University of California, Los Angeles, and after a year of residency in pediatrics at Johns Hopkins, I entered the field of radiology. I took my radiology training at U.C.L.A., the U.S. Public Health Service, and Johns Hopkins Hospital.

I started practice with a radiology group in Baltimore. I later changed to the Patuxent Medical Group (PMG), a multi-specialty medical practice that provided the medical care for the Columbia Medicine Plan, an HMO. I stayed for more than 27 years until my recent retirement. This group was owned by BlueCross/ BlueShield of Maryland for the last 18 years I was in practice.

During my tenure, I became the medical administrator and played a variety of management roles in PMG, including Medical Director and President. These roles and the fact that the group was owned by BlueCross/BlueShield opened new doors for me, and I began performing additional work as an insurance administrator. This included being a Senior Vice-President for BlueCross/BlueShield of Maryland and President of their then four HMOs. I did not plan this career path; it was a process of evolution.

Like everyone else, from time to time, I encountered my own medical problems, and, whether I liked it or not, I became a patient. I truly learned what it is like to be a patient, however, when I came face-to-face with the diagnosis of a life-threatening illness. I broke one of my personal rules on being a patient: **Never be a great case of anything!**

HERE'S WHAT HAPPENED...

I was bothered with ringing in my ears, a condition known as tinnitus, so I went to see my Ear, Nose, and Throat doctor. He scheduled a Magnetic Resonance Imaging study, commonly known as an MRI. This is like a sophisticated x-ray of the brain. The nerves to my ears were fine, but the test found "something" in the right side of my brain.

Because I am a radiologist, my doctors invited me to review the results with them. As I walked into the reading room with my wife, I remember pointing to a study on one of the view boxes and saying, "Boy, am I glad those aren't mine!" There was an obvious mass in the right parietal lobe (upper right side) of the patient's brain. I was shocked to find out that this patient was indeed me.

To say that I was devastated is a complete understatement of my emotional state at that moment. The initial review of the MRI led to the conclusion that I had an aggressive brain tumor and probably had 6 months or less to live.

That night, my wife and I had dinner with our 34-year-old daughter (my other two children were out of town). The discussion revolved around wills and final wishes. The next day, I was scheduled to have a CT scan to get a better picture of the mass. This study again showed a mass but some of its features were less ominous than on the MRI. The films were reviewed by two professors at a top medical school who concluded that I most likely had a cancer that had spread (metastasized) to my brain, quite possibly a malignant melanoma, the deadliest form of skin cancer. You can just imagine the mental state my family and I were in by this time!

Next I met with a neurologist who examined me for any clinical signs of a tumor. He believed some of the findings did not fit the typical brain tumor, and that the lesion might not be "as aggressive" as the previous doctors had determined.

He referred me to a neurosurgeon, the next logcial step in the treatment process. I chose a senior neurosurgeon at a teaching hospital because of the conflicting opinions I had already received and because of the potential severity of the abnormality. After reviewing my studies, he said the mass was something that most neurosurgeons would operate on, and if I desired, he would do so. However, he agreed with my neurologist that there were some aspects that didn't fit the usual presentation of a malignant brain tumor. He said that it could just as possibly be a benign mass and suggested we do nothing but monitor it closely. I knew enough about medicine and had enough confidence in my doctor's judgment that I did not get a second neurosurgical opinion.

Because I knew how to manage the medical system—and as I will teach you in this book—I received rapid care with very minimal delay. Nonetheless, those few days were an extremely anxious time for me and my family.

If I hadn't the knowledge to expedite my own care, it is most likely that this entire scenario would have played out over the course of several weeks instead of a few days. The anxiety over something like this could be overwhelming. Now, after 4 years, one CT scan, ten MRIs, and multiple diagnoses later, no doctor is yet certain what this mass is that is in my head—a classic example that proves that medicine is really an art, not a science. (I will get more into this discussion later.) My diagnoses to date include: a variety of tumors, both benign and malignant; a mass of scar tissue from an old injury; and a mass remaining from a prior infection, possibly from some type of parasite. But it's still there, though it isn't changing, and the longer it is stable, the better it is. Therefore, we are pursuing the watch-and-wait approach.

By the way, the tinnitus that first brought me to the doctor in the first place turned out to be unrelated to the mass and required no treatment.

JUST IN CASE I DIDN'T GET MY FILL OF ANXIETY FROM THIS FIRST EXPERIENCE, I RECENTLY HAD ANOTHER MEDICAL ADVENTURE...

I had gone to my doctor for a routine physical. He did appropriate blood tests for my age and the medications I was taking. He found two of my liver enzyme tests were high and stayed high on a repeat test. So, he suggested I get an ultrasound (sonogram) of my liver. This study showed some fatty changes in my liver that aren't supposed to be there. The doctor and I discussed what diagnosis this might suggest in view of my general health and lifestyle. Some of the possibilities were not very pleasant.

One very possible theory was that it was caused by my excessive sugar habit driving my blood insulin too high, too often. Other possibilities included Hepatitis C, a serious infectious disease that can lead to cirrhosis of the liver. Not only was I stressed about my own diagnosis, the possibility that I had an infectious disease like Hepatitis C that I could have given to my wife was extremely upsetting. Your own health is hard enough to contemplate, but in truth few of us live in a vacuum, and many of our health problems have significant impact and possibly even risks for those we love.

He suggested that I change my diet, keep up my exercise program, and come back for more lab studies in 6 weeks. Basically, I had to give up sugar and all foods that the body can rapidly convert to sugar. This meant no desserts to a man who had been a chocoholic for his entire life. It also meant only whole-grain or stone-ground breads, brown rice instead of white rice, sweet potatoes instead of white potatoes, and no foods with more than a minimal amount of sugar. My dessert affair was over!

I complied rigidly with the diet (it is amazing what the fear of significant illness can do to you), and my follow-up

1

lab studies showed remarkable improvement. The good news is that this does appear to be a condition that I can manage with diet. The bad news is that I have to follow it for the rest of my life.

Through these experiences, **I learned firsthand the challenges of being a patient in a medical maze of differing opinions,** cold hospital rooms (and sometimes cold people!), and the avalanche of insurance forms and procedures. I also realized how difficult it was to get the care I needed, even with all my experience and skills as a physician and a medical manager. Through it all, I kept wondering how someone without my background and knowledge could find their way though the medical system. I believe I bring a level of empathy to this book that I hope you can feel.

> I experienced firsthand how hard it is to get the care you need when you need it and what it feels like when doctors are not sure what is wrong.

How I Became a Medical Mentor

Helping people get the medical care they need when they need it began one patient at a time. I would often work with my wife, who is a psychotherapist with some 30 years' experience, to help family and friends with their medical-care problems. This began as what I call a translating function.

Friends and acquaintances would call and tell me what their doctors had said, and I would translate it into plain English. Gradually, this began to evolve into helping people with the strategies necessary to obtain the care they wanted. I came to realize that there is a greater need to help people navigate the medical system than my wife and I could personally provide. I also came to realize that helping others navigate this medical system gave me a great amount of satisfaction. Now, as a 63-year-old retired physician, it is my professional passion and my avocation.

> Many patients lack the knowledge needed to succeed as a patient in the medical and insurance systems. I have that knowledge and will teach you how to be your own medical advocate.

I continue to encounter people who feel confused and frustrated when dealing with their doctors and insurance companies. **They don't have the special knowledge needed today to succeed as a patient. I have that knowledge and wish to share it so you can learn to be your own medical advocate and get the care you need in the most direct way.** Let me guide you and I will empower you to comfortably and successfully navigate your own way through the health-care system.

During the years since I began practicing medicine, I have seen a tremendous transition. For example, the Columbia Medical Plan, which was one of the finest HMOs in the country (named fourth in the nation and first in Maryland two years in a row by the *U.S. News and World Report* survey), has been closed. What does it mean to medicine when a medical plan of that quality is shut down? What has happened is that the whole nature of managed care and medicine itself has changed. The relationship between the doctor and the insurance company has changed with it. As a result, unfortunately, **the relationships between patients and doctors and their insurance companies also changed.**

Medicine for the patient of today reminds me of the story of the group of blind men trying to describe an elephant. One has hold of the trunk, one grabs a leg, one is feeling the mammoth side of the animal, one has a hand on a tusk, and one has the tail. Each has a valid experience, but alone each experiences a completely different animal. Medicine is a lot like that. Hopefully, by the end of this book, you will have gained the ability to see the whole animal. In so doing, you should be better prepared to gain the care you need from the system.

Key Take Home Messages

- The health-care system in America is a mess, and it is not going to get better anytime soon.

- The relationships between patients and doctors and patients and insurance companies have changed—and none of them are happy about it.

- It takes insider's knowledge and self-empowerment to be your own medical advocate so you can get the care you need and deserve.

- The approach and the skills to do this are easy to learn.

- Sometimes you need to be more aggressive in your approach to get what you need out of the medical system.

WHO'S IN CHARGE
HERE ANYWAY?

Is it really important who's in charge
of my health care?

What do I do if my doctor doesn't want
to partner with me?

Should my doctor be board-certified?

How can I assess the quality of my doctor?

Should I choose a young doctor right out
of training or an older, more-experienced doctor?

How do I tell my doctor that I am leaving
her practice?

Whose time is more valuable—
mine or my doctor's?

Who is the one person who should
be in charge?

You Have Options

Your medical care and the decisions surrounding it can take several forms.

> FOR INSTANCE. . .
> You are waiting in the exam room, and in walks the doctor, wearing a long white coat, stethoscope around her neck, and an aura of invincibility over her whole being. You sit there quietly in your partially torn (they always seem to be) paper gown, trying to look dignified. She asks a few questions, pokes here, prods there, and then pauses for a moment to think to herself. Finally, she tells you your diagnosis, and what you are to do. You say "thank you," and go and do as you're told.

This is the classic paternalistic style of medicine in which the doctor determines the problem, makes the decision as to what should be done about it, and the patient accepts it without question. This is the Dr. Welby image of medicine which, if you're old enough, you used to see on television—the kindly, wise general practitioner who brings you into the world and then guides you through all your illnesses. Somehow, she always knows just what you need in order to get you well, and you have blind faith that she is always right.

Nice picture, but not very true! The assumption that the doctor is always right is as old-fashioned as Dr. Welby. This assumption has been reinforced by the growing belief in the ultimate power of science, and the lost appreciation for the critical role of subjective human decision making that is critical to medicine. Ironically, the progress that has been made in medical science is the reason this type of doctor-patient relationship no longer works to the patient's benefit.

Let me clear this up for anyone who has any delusions: **Medicine is an art!** Medicine is based in science, but there is a great range of subjectivity when it comes to making a diagnosis and deciding the best treatment. This subjectivity is what makes practicing medicine an art. A doctor's actual certainty in her decisions can range from 99-plus percent in the best case to a hunch that may be a little better than 50-50. This is not a bad thing, but it is the reality.

For example, my personal experience that I described in chapter 1 put me in the hunch category. It was clear that my tests and findings could be interpreted in more than one way. The art of medicine is the physician drawing on her experience to evaluate the various findings and conclude what she believes to be the most likely diagnosis. Deciding what the next step should be is also—and possibly the most important—part of her art. My neurosurgeon told me that there would be no problem finding a neurosurgeon who would operate, based on the tests that had been done. Yet with the same data and based on his evaluation of them, and his own personal experience, he recommended not to operate.

This is the art of medicine. If medicine were a pure science, a given set of data would lead all practitioners to the same conclusion. The ideal of Dr. Welby is as fictional as the show.

The fact that medicine is an art is what's wrong with the paternalistic system. How do you know where the physician is on her spectrum of certainty? If you just accept everything she says, sometimes you'll do great and sometimes you won't. The paternalistic system does not include discussion and the give and take necessary for you to understand how much confidence she has in her recommendations, nor does it include you in the decision-making process.

AN ALTERNATIVE INTERACTION IS...
You are waiting in the exam room and in walks the doctor. She sits down and updates you on the results of recent tests you had done. She then suggests the next step in your care and asks you how you feel about it. You respond by pulling out an article you printed out from the Internet. You say that this is the approach you want to take. When the doctor wants to discuss it, you say you don't. You have spoken with friends, researched the Internet, and participated in chat rooms. Your mind is made up, and you expect the doctor to follow your plan. When she raises concerns about your proposed course of treatment, you tell her you are the patient and this is what you want to do. End of discussion.

This scenario is where the patient dominates all decisions. This is the new Internet-savvy patient who looks up every test and diagnosis, takes it as gospel, and depends solely on it to make a decision about what should be done and when. If the doctor disagrees, the patient pulls out the latest article relevant to the topic at hand. The problem with this system is the word "dominates." The average patient can not possibly bring to the decision the depth of experience and understanding that the physician can. Even if the patient is also a doctor and has the knowledge base, in my experience the doctor-as-patient won't have the emotional distance necessary for rational decision making.

I will get into the pros and cons of using the Internet for medical research in chapter 17, but for now the issue is: Who should be the decision-maker? Suffice it to say that the patient who is dominating the decision making is heading for real trouble.

> A THIRD STORY LINE STARTS MUCH
> LINE THE SECOND...
> You are waiting in the exam room and in walks the doctor. She sits down and updates you on the results of recent tests you had done. She then suggests the next step in your care and asks you how you feel about it. You respond by asking questions about the test results. You ask why she is making her recommendation. She takes your response seriously, answers your questions directly, and then asks if you are ready to proceed with her proposed care plan. If you are, great. If not, she asks what further reservations you have and how the two of you can reach a mutual decision.

This is a **partnership**. Both the patient and the physician work together as equal partners to guide the medical course. This requires some mutual understanding on the part of both parties. They both have to be in tune to the concept of sharing the decision making. The patient must feel free to ask all the questions she wants, and the doctor has to be willing to consider them seriously and answer them fully. This can be challenging for both parties, but it is worth it. It can happen by accident or just

2

evolve, but I believe a direct conversation between doctor and patient about how health-care decisions will be made works well.

Either the doctor or the patient can establish this as the relationship style, but be prepared to take the first step. For example, when your doctor suggests a test, makes a diagnosis, or brings up any issue concerning your health, say something like, "Can you share your thoughts and logic behind this recommendation with me so we can decide together what's best for me?" It may take one or two passes at this to get your doctor to connect, but I think you'll be amazed at how responsive she will be.

> To successfully be your own medical advocate, you want to establish a partnership with your doctor and share control of your health-care decision.

- **Is it really important who's in charge of my health care?**
  The answer is an emphatic yes. **This decision may be the most important medical decision you make.** So I submit that you should care quite a bit. You may never have thought about it, but take a moment to do so now. Do you want to be doing what you are told based on someone else's assumption of your best interest? Do you want to be making decisions you are not qualified to make? Or, do you want to be partnering with someone who has greater knowledge and experience in this area and can guide you and be your consultant?

  You know what personal values you hold most dear. You know your own wants and fears. If you can honestly share them with your medical partner, you will be amazed by how good you will feel about the results.

  I believe most doctors today welcome the opportunity to partner with their patients. They may not always know how to take the first step, but they do care that you are a part of the process. It would be great if your doctor raised the issue directly and opened a discussion on the decision-making process. But, if she doesn't, then it is in your best interest to initiate the process. If you have selected the right doctor, you will find that she is readily open to this type of partnership. **Do not be shy or hesitant about initiating the conversation.** Don't forget, it is your body and your health we are talking about. You want help understanding what is happening and in processing the data.

The key to this type of relationship is you. And the word to keep on the tip of your tongue is *why*. **There is no instance in which you are not justified in asking your physician the rationale behind her recommendation or decision.** If she says the decision is up to you, say, "I know, but one of the things I weigh is what you think is best. I want to take your recommendation into account as I make my decision."

It's a Two-Way Relationship

The doctor's role in your partnership is to advise and inform you. It is also to support your decision, unless she feels that your decision requires unethical, illegal, or medically unacceptable care. In that case, she should share her reservations with you. If she cannot convince you to change your decision, then she should be willing to help you find another physician or an alternative practitioner who may be able to support you in the path you want to take. This is partnering. You will see how amazingly easy it is for a decision to be reached when both patient and doctor feel good about working together as a team.

- **What do I do if my doctor doesn't want to partner with me?**

  I am not a big fan of changing doctors. It is obviously too hard to find a good doctor who is taking new patients and to work out good communications and a trusting relationship with that doctor. However, if you cannot establish this type of relationship with your current doctor, you may have to change doctors. In other words, if your doctor won't meet you halfway in managing your medical concerns, then you can't afford to be her patient.

> If your doctor won't be your
> partner in your medical care, then
> you can't afford to be her patient!

2

How to Find a New Doctor

One of the questions I am frequently asked is how to choose a doctor. There are many resources you can use to help you in this process. Possibly the most common thing that many people find helpful is to **ask family members or friends** for their recommendations. **If you know any doctors or other people in the medical field,** they often are a great source of referrals. While they may be hesitant to say that one doctor is better than another, an easy approach is to ask them who they go to for their medical care. If you ask several people and the same name keeps being mentioned, this is a good sign that the doctor is well-respected.

Think about the qualities that are important to you in a doctor, and try to find out if the doctor you are considering has them. For instance, is she good at returning telephone calls, does she offer evening or weekend hours, and so on.

> There are a variety of resources
> you can access to find the names
> of potential doctors. I prefer those
> in which you have a personal
> level of trust with the person
> making the referral.

You can check out a doctor recommendation or start your **search for a physician by contacting the physician referral service at either your local hospital** or your local medical society. This, however, has its limitations. These resources can give you some information about the doctor's specialty and training, but I have never known any of them to comment on the quality of the doctor. The doctors are usually placed on their referral lists by either having privileges in that hospital or belonging to that medical society.

Some medical practices now advertise their services. Listing a practice in the telephone book is a long-standing approach used by many doctors and is usually considered to be helpful even to their established patients. Advertising in the newspaper or on the radio is a more recent phenomenon. Some patients have mixed feelings about this, and I leave it to you to decide if this is a positive or negative. I am not aware of any research relating advertising to medical quality.

Once you have accomplished this search and found your potential choice, **make sure that the doctor is in your insurance network** (this is discussed in detail in chapter 21). Also, check with her office to be sure that she is accepting new patients.

• Should my doctor be board-certified?

Board certification is verification that your doctor has accomplished a certain level of training and proficiency in the specialty she practices. In most specialties, this is becoming an expected accomplishment. The American Board of Medical Specialties (ABMS), an arm of the American Medical Association, is responsible for establishing and regulating the approved specialty boards. The ABMS has a web site (**www.abms.org**) where you can look up a doctor to find out if she is board-certified in the specialty you are seeking.

If she is, it is confirmation that the doctor has at least a baseline level of training and proficiency in a specialty. If she is not, you want to discuss why with your doctor. If you have not yet met the prospective doctor, you may want to discuss this concern with the person referring you to the new doctor. Alternatively, you may want to eliminate any doctor from consideration unless she has board certification in the appropriate specialty. Remember, board certification is a measure of training and competency at the completion of training. It is not the total measure of quality.

• How can I assess the quality of my doctor?

Some people want to know more about a potential doctor than her board-certification status. There are some Internet websites that you can use to help you find certain information about a physician. A good place to start is your **state medical board.** These boards go by different names in different states, but they have a common responsibility for licensing and supervising the medical care provided by physicians in that state. You can find the website for the medical board in your state by accessing **www.docboard.org**. The data available varies from state to state, but you can frequently find information about a doctor's training, specialty, and a variety of potentially important facts, such as any history of medical disciplinary actions, malpractice judgments, and felony convictions, among others.

If your potential physician takes Medicare patients, you can check out the web site **www.medicare.gov**. Information on patient satisfaction with the physician's practice and/or Medicare health plan can be found here by looking for the **Consumer Assessment of Health Plan Survey (CHAPS)** report. If you have difficulty linking to the survey, try searching for the survey by name on whichever search engine you use. The www.medicare.gov site is also a resource for other information about both physician practices and different types of health plans for Medicare patients.

> There are reputable web sites that can provide you with some educational and background information on the doctor you are considering.

- **Should I choose a young doctor right out of training or an older, more-experienced doctor?**
  Over the years, there have been some interesting scientific papers written that attempt to relate the age and experience of a doctor to the quality of medical care. The conclusions have been somewhat mixed. More recently, researchers reviewed a large number of these scientific articles to assess common findings and trends. They found that older physicians who have been in practice longer may not be providing as high-quality care as younger physicians who are more recently trained. The difference seemed to center around knowledge of newer medical techniques. Keep in mind that this conclusion was based on averages and does not necessarily apply to individuals. **Your key concern should be whether an older physician is staying up with the latest advances in medicine.**

My opinion is that you want a physician who is caring, intelligent, well-trained, and stays current in her field. Of course, this is subjective and will be the hard to assess, but they are things worth asking about when looking for physician referrals.

> IN MY OWN SPECIALTY...
> The best radiologist I ever knew, Dr. Leo Rigler, was 83 years old when we first met. He had had a brilliant academic career and made some of the fundamental discoveries in chest radiology. He stayed current on the latest scientific literature throughout his life. When anyone discussed a case with him, you were able to hear a combination of the best that the science of medicine had to offer (knowledge of the scientific literature) with the best that the art of medicine had to offer (experience and good judgment).

Therefore, I would say that what you should be looking for is a physician who is both well-trained and diligent in keeping up with the developments in her specialty. If she has years of experience behind her, all the better. If she has the experience but you have reason to believe she is not working to stay current with the latest medical developments, then you have reason to be concerned.

> The age of your doctor isn't as important as finding one who is caring, intelligent, well-trained, and stays current in her field.

- **How do I tell my doctor that I am leaving her practice?**
  After you have selected a new doctor, notify your current doctor's office that you will be making this change. Remember, **you have the right to change doctors.** Even if you are leaving because you are dissatisfied with the care you are getting, you should not act angry or make accusations. In fact, I would advise you to **do it in the most positive manner possible.** You do not have to do it face-to-face. You can call the office and notify the office staff.
  You do want to have your medical records transferred to

your new doctor's office. The original records are the legal property of the doctor. **In most states, you do have the right to have a copy of your medical records transferred to another doctor.** You may also have the right to have your own copy of your medical records. The office may charge you a copying fee, but that varies from office to office. Again let me stress that you want to manage the transfer in a positive fashion. You never know when you may cross paths with your former doctor again. A little care to be positive now may pay major dividends later.

> Changing doctors requires some thoughtfulness. Try to make it a positive experience for everyone involved.

- **Whose time is more valuable—mine or my doctor's?**
  Both your time and your doctor's time are valuable. Patients often have to take time off from work, arrange child care, or make other scheduling adjustments to fit the doctor's schedule. So you want to be on time for your appointments. On the other hand, the doctor has a responsibility to not keep you waiting. The reality of medicine is that sometimes patients arrive for an appointment and are sicker than expected and take up more time than was scheduled. So, the doctor gets behind in her schedule. **The doctor should have her staff tell you if a wait has developed.** It is also fair for you to be able to ask this question when you arrive for your appointment.

  WHAT IS NOT FAIR IS...
  A doctor I know put up a sign in his office that said, "If you are more than 15 minutes late for your appointment, we will have to reschedule you for another time."

  Now this doctor on occasion will run behind, sometimes by 45 minutes, because of unexpected problems with other patients. However, if a doctor expects you to wait when the schedule doesn't work as expected, you have the right to expect the same courtesy in return.

> Your time is just as valuable
> as your doctor's. Don't allow her
> to think otherwise.

Who's *Not* in Charge of Your Health Care

Your insurance company should not be in charge of your health care. Depending on the type of insurance you have, there may be more or less "management" of your care through the policies and procedures of your insurance company. You really need to understand what that insurance management is. You do not want to let your insurance company limit the decisions you want to make concerning your care.

Medical insurance is a contract between you and your insurance company that usually says they will pay for your medical care under certain conditions (the insurance benefit package). Insurance packages vary widely. Often times, they vary by what your employer picks for you (if your insurance is through your work). I know the benefit books the insurance companies provide often look quite daunting, but it is worth the time it takes to understand your benefits. We will discuss later how to work with your insurance company if you are trying to obtain a service that is not usually covered.

> Your insurance company is not in
> charge of your medical care.

- **Who is the one person who should be in charge?**
  In the end, yes—you, the wise patient advocate. **You must have the final word.** But keep in mind that a wise voice is an informed voice. Are there other voices you should hear? Absolutely!

  First there is your physician partner. Usually there are family and friends with whom you will discuss your care. If they are skilled listeners, they will help you to sort out your thoughts. Sometimes, well-meaning people will want to "help" by telling you medical horror stories about people they knew in similar situations and the disastrous things that happened to them. Stop the conversation! But, as we will discuss later, a trusted family member or friend can be absolutely essential as a second set of ears for you as you talk to your doctor. They can't make your decisions for you, but they can be invaluable in making sure you have the facts straight. In the end, the final decision is yours.

2

Key Take Home Messages

- It matters very much who is in charge of your health care.

- The best relationship is one in which you and your doctor have a partnership and share control of your health care.

- Your doctor-partner will not only give you the time you need to get all your questions answered, but she will encourage you to ask questions.

- If your doctor won't take the time to be your partner, then you can't afford to be her patient!

- Changing doctors should be a careful and thoughtful process, but there are many resources you can look to for help.

- Your insurance company is not in charge of your health care.

- In the end, the informed patient advocate makes the final decision.

3

THE DOCTOR'S OFFICE—THE ART OF THE APPOINTMENT

What happens if the office staff is rude?

What if my doctor doesn't have time
to address all my concerns?

Do I have to accept unnecessary delays?

The office can't find the referral,
and I forgot my copy!

The Hub of Your Medical Care

Doctors' offices are busy places. All told, Americans make an estimated 890 million office visits a year. That averages to three visits for every man, woman, and child—including the 9 percent of adults and 10 percent of children who don't go at all.

Most of your health-care needs throughout life will be centered in the doctor's office. Obviously, the number of visits per year varies by age, generally rising with age. In addition, women tend to make more visits than men. (There are only two age groups in which male visits are higher: under 15 and over 75).

The office of your **primary-care physician is where most medical discussions take place** and decisions are made. If you need care from another doctor, this is where you get the referral. If you need surgery, tests, or other procedures, this is where they are scheduled. It is the hub of your medical care—or at least it should be. For all these reasons, it is important that you have your best medical relationship with your primary-care physician.

Walking through the Door

When you walk through the door, you want to feel welcome and safe. Your visits should be positive and productive. As your own proactive medical advocate, you need to have a strategy to make sure you get what you want from each doctor's visit.

There are at least two things that can impede this process. One, I believe most of us usually feel some degree of anxiety when entering the doctor's office. Two, the doctor's staff is often considered an impediment to our care, rather than caring people who want to help us get the care we desire.

A VISIT AT ITS WORST CAN EVOLVE AS SADLY AS THIS
EXAMPLE I HAVE SEEN MANY TIMES...
The patient approaches the reception counter to check in. When the front office staff does not respond soon enough (in the patient's mind), he raises his voice and is rude and borderline abusive about the staff's lack of attention. When brought back to the exam room by the doctor's health

assistant, the patient is better behaved but still somewhat hostile and rude. When the doctor comes in the room, the patient is all smiles and appreciative. What's wrong with this picture?

3

This type of encounter, I believe, often is due to the patient's unrecognized anxiety and a lack of trust in the good intentions of the staff. I don't believe every patient feels this way, and those who do feel it to varying degrees. Many are not aware of it. The importance of this example is that if you behave in this manner, you lower your chances of achieving what you want from the visit. Even though this patient behaves well with the doctor, the fact that he antagonizes the front-desk and back-office staff will get back to him, undermining the patient/doctor relationship. So, what can you do to lessen your anxiety and make your visit more pleasant and productive?

Think of your doctor's office as a team. You want all the team members pulling for you, even when you are perfectly well. You want the front desk to be eager to accommodate you and get you the most convenient appointment. You want the billing staff to make sure your bill is correct so you are not bogged down later in paperwork from your insurance company or from your doctor's billing company. You want the back-office health assistant to be glad to see you. The genuine warmth and caring that you will receive when this relationship is healthy is a real comfort when you are feeling anxious. And, of course, you want your doctor to consider you a patient that he can work with in a positive way to resolve your medical needs.

> Your partnership with your doctor includes every member of his office team.

You achieve quality relationships by intentionally developing them. I do not suggest that you be false or "butter up" the staff. Rather, let your true, kind nature through. If you are feeling good, say so. If you are feeling lousy, share that too. But you might also share how glad you are to be in the doctor's office to get some help.

Staff most often choose to work in a doctor's office because they want to help people. They are caregivers in the best sense. Let them help you. It will make both of you feel good, and form the basis of a solid relationship. By the way, don't be afraid to tell the staff if you are having anxiety over the visit. You might be pleasantly surprised that many will respond by taking extra measures to make you comfortable and less anxious.

- **What happens if the office staff is rude?**

Sadly, the pressure of a busy office sometimes can make staff behave badly. I suggest you first try to talk to those involved about how you perceive they are treating you. Do this in a rational, not confrontational, manner. This means, don't accuse. For example, don't say: "You are being rude for no reason." Rather, say, "You seem angry to me. Did I do something to offend you?"

Of course, if you are not feeling well, your patience can wear thin. If you make no progress, ask to speak to the office manager. Most doctors' offices have someone designated as the manager who is responsible for ensuring that the office runs smoothly. If you can not resolve it at this level, then bring it up when you see your doctor. Approach it in as positive a way as possible. For example, you might say to your doctor, "I have been trying to create a positive relationship with your office staff, but it is not happening. I have received several rude comments at the front desk. I have discussed it with the staff and with your office manager, but the rudeness continues. Can you help me solve this problem?"

You may think that you're wasting the doctor's time but you are not. In my experience, doctors who receive this type of feedback from their patients work to reach a positive outcome. **Doctors have no practice without you, the patient.** Most doctors I know want satisfied patients and want their staffs to do their part to produce that result.

If the problem persists, get back to your doctor and tell him so. Patients I have mentored who can not resolve this type of problem eventually change doctors. Before you do so, however, tell your doctor that you will be forced to leave his practice if things do not change.

Planning Your Visit

The successful health advocate goes to the doctor's office prepared. That calls for a plan. The first thing you want to do is to **make an up-to-date list of the medicines you are taking, including the dosages**. This should include prescription medicines as well as over-the-counter medicines, vitamins, and other supplements.

3

> **SOMETHING IMPORTANT FOR YOUR WALLET.** It is a good habit to always carry a copy of your "current medications" list with you. You never know when an illness or accident might occur, and having this list on your person could prove important, even life-saving. I keep my list on a small card the size of a credit card and carry it in my wallet. When my medicines change, I update my card. It is also a good idea to make sure that the important people in your life know where you keep your list and have a copy of the list, too. If you are injured, you may not be able to give this information to your medical caregivers, while those close to you will.

Check if any of your prescriptions are about to run out. While you are at the doctor's office, you might as well get the refills you need and save a phone call or another trip to the office. If you are planning a vacation soon, make sure you have enough medicines to cover you while you are away.

Also, think of all the questions you have about your health since your last visit, even minor health issues. Write them down—and do not forget to take this list with you! Check the list carefully while you are with your doctor to make sure you get all your questions answered. There are few things more frustrating than walking out of an appointment and 30 minutes later thinking, "I meant to ask him that while I was there!"

If you are having a problem with bills from your insurance company or from the doctor's office, take them with you. When you check in at the front desk, ask to speak to someone about them. If you have billing issues, it is a good idea to arrive for your appointment early, so you have time to deal with them prior to seeing the doctor.

> Plan ahead for your visit—
> take a list of your medications
> and a list of your current
> health concerns.

- **What if my doctor doesn't have time to address all my concerns?**

  I have discussed my approach of preparing a list of questions with several of my primary-care partners. I was surprised that some expressed concern that the patient would have a list of issues longer than could possibly be answered in the time scheduled for the appointment. Doctors' offices generally allow 15 to 20 minutes for a routine visit. This doesn't mean you should not bring a list or that you should limit your list. It means you need to **make an appointment that allows enough time to discuss your entire list.** Therefore, if you have multiple issues to discuss with your doctor, you need to tell the office staff when you schedule the appointment. Even if it is a special visit to discuss a current problem, you should feel entitled to address other concerns you may have.

  You need to be specific about needing more time. If you find after you have scheduled the appointment that your list is growing, call the office and discuss it with the staff; otherwise, you may have to return for a second appointment.

  If the staff tells you that the doctor can only see you for an allotted amount of time because of insurance company policy— don't buy it! If you do your part by letting the office know as early as possible that you have multiple issues, **he can give you the time you need if he chooses.**

  Let me warn you that this may not always work at first. If the office will not give you the extra time, despite your best (and positively made) efforts, take your list and bring up all your concerns anyway. If you have done as I have advised, and your doctor says there is not enough time to discuss your whole list, explain to him how you communicated your need for extra time to his office staff. Don't forget, you are in a partnership with your doctor to provide you with the best health care possible. Only by letting him know things are not going right can he change procedures to provide it to you in the most efficient manner.

As we go through this book together, you will find again and again how important it is for you to not accept less than you deserve and need.

> I KNOW A PATIENT WHO WENT INTO HIS DOCTOR'S OFFICE AND SAW A SIGN THAT SAID...
> "If you are here for a routine health checkup, no questions about illnesses are allowed."

> I KNOW ANOTHER PATIENT WHO WENT INTO HIS DOCTOR'S OFFICE AND SAW A SIGN THAT SAID...
> "Only two questions can be discussed with the doctor in any one office visit."

There are also other signals that say your doctor does not have time for you. One is the newer trend of being seen by a nurse practitioner or a certified physician's assistant when you show up for an appointment you thought was with your doctor. It is likely that these people will have more time to spend with you. Some doctors' offices may try to schedule you with another doctor in the practice. However, this should not mean you can not see your own doctor if you want. If this is a pattern in your doctor's office, talk to him about it. Also, specify your preference when you make your appointment.

> Your doctor does have time for you! Just let the staff know that you need extra time in advance of your visit.

• Do I have to accept unnecessary delays?

One of the key skills you need to develop is how to avoid unnecessary delays when you need to see or get in touch with your doctor. Delays come in many forms. The most frequent is what is commonly called telephone tag. You call your doctor, he is not available, you leave a message, he calls you back, you are not available, and he leaves a message. This cycle can go on for days!

You should tell the office staff what you want to talk to the doctor about. When you make the first call, find out from the office when the doctor will be available to receive calls and make an appointment to call back. Or, find out a timeframe when you can expect the doctor to call back so you can make sure that you are available to take the call.

If you still can't get through to your doctor, your next approach depends on the situation. If you still need a question answered right away by your doctor, and he isn't calling you back, then ask the office for an appointment for that day to see the doctor.

One of the financial facts of a medical practice is that doctors don't get paid for advice they give out or the time they spend on the telephone. They only get paid when they see the patient. It seems to me that, for some doctors, this is creating a pattern of limiting the amount of telephone time they are taking with patients. So, if you want to talk to your doctor and he won't call back, make an appointment to see him face-to-face. Be clear how urgent the problem is so the office can look for an opening in the proper timeframe.

If you need an appointment and can't get one, I suggest you go into the office in person and ask the office staff what you should do. I suggest that you specifically say, "I can't get an appointment...what should I do?" If they tell you that there is no solution, then **I suggest one of two strategies**:

If you want to still work with this doctor, tell the staff you are going to sit down in the waiting room and wait until the doctor will talk to you. Be prepared to stay awhile if you say this. I suggest you bring a book and start reading it. This will let the staff know that you are there to stay until the office responds. I know patients who have done this, and the result is usually that it doesn't take long before you get to see the doctor, or a telephone appointment with the doctor is arranged.

If you conclude that this is not the right doctor for your needs, ask the office staff to begin copying your medical records, as you will be calling them with the name of your new doctor. **Remember, even the world's best doctor is no good to you if you can't get to him when you need him!**

> There are strategies that will let you talk to or see your doctor when you need to—including right now.

3

Other unnecessary delays can happen when you need to schedule an urgent appointment as well as a follow-up appointment. It is amazing how **weeks can be added to the evaluation and treatment of a medical problem because of booking issues**. You can often speed this up by taking the first available appointment. Let me say, having a health problem can cause a major disruption in your routine. Most of us try to limit the inconvenience by getting an ideal appointment time. This is fine when you have a need to see the doctor that is not urgent. However, if you are acutely ill or worried that there might be something seriously wrong with you, you want to be seen as soon as possible. The same holds true for follow-up visits; you want to get to the conclusion or the next step as soon as possible. This may mean moving things around on your calendar to do so. I know this may sound like the logical thing to do, but I have seen many patients experience unnecessary delays in getting needed health care because they'd rather wait for the ideal appointment time.

> You can avoid delays by being flexible on the appointment times you accept.

Getting a Referral

Your primary-care provider (PCP)—be it a family practitioner, internist, or, in the case of a child, a pediatrician—is home base for all your medical care. You want to be sure that your primary doctor is always up-to-date on your medical care, even if it is provided by a specialist.

If you have a managed-care insurance plan, you may need a referral to see a specialist. (This is something you need to know about your insurance policy. If you are not sure, see chapters 21 and 22, about understanding your insurance policy and its referral process.) If so, get your referral from your primary-care physician at the time of your visit. Frequently, because of the way some insurance policies operate, your doctor may have to get an authorization from the insurance company before he can complete the referral. In that case, you may not want to wait in his office as it may take a few hours while the paperwork is completed. PCP's will frequently fax the referral form directly to the specialist. However, you want to make sure that you have a copy of the completed referral form in your hands to take with you to the specialist. The referral is your verification that you have an appointment.

It is unfortunate, but it is common for someone to show up for an appointment with a specialist and discover that the **specialist's office can't find the referral form and will not see the patient without it**. As long as you have a copy, no problem. In my experience, this also commonly happens when you are being referred to a hospital for testing. You save yourself a great deal of frustration in these instances when you can simply hand the staff a copy of the referral.

In defense of the office or hospital staff, the current insurance environment creates a flood of paperwork. They are trying to keep track of it all, but they frequently find it overwhelming. This is an instance where you can help them and speed up your own care.

> Understanding the referral process is a key skill to navigating the health-care system.

- **The office can't find the referral, and I forgot my copy!**
First, don't panic. Second, do not let them cancel your appointment or send you back to your PCP to get a new referral. Ask the staff to call your PCP and have a copy of the referral faxed to the specialist. This can all take place while you are waiting to see the doctor. If the staff says they can not do it,

ask to use their telephone, or use your cell phone, so you can call yourself. Believe me, you will not be the first patient that this ever happened to.

If the staff is busy and is resistant to your request, this is one of the times when you need to get assertive. Of course, you can avoid it all if you make sure to take a copy of the referral with you.

3

Cancellations and No-Shows
"I forgot to go to the doctor!"

It's happened to all of us. Whether you totally forgot about your appointment and became a "no-show," or had a conflict and needed to cancel at the last minute, make sure you follow up.

If you totally forgot and did not call to cancel, you need to do two things. Call to apologize and also to reschedule your appointment. Not showing up for an appointment, no matter how unintentional, is rude. As your part of the partnership, you should acknowledge it with a call to the office. Rescheduling is important because you don't want to ignore a follow-up or routine visit, and you can't expect the doctor's office to contact you with a reminder.

If you missed the appointment because your reason to see the doctor resolved itself, you still need to contact the office and let them know that you are not rescheduling. Keep communication honest and open on all levels.

Key Take Home Messages

- Your primary-care physician's office is the hub of your medical care.

- Make sure your doctor has an up-to-date record of all your medications and any visits to the Emergency Room, specialists, or any other medical care you have received since you last saw him.

- Come prepared for your visit—make a list of your concerns and check your medications to see if you need prescription renewals.

- Don't accept unnecessary delays in getting an appointment when you need to see your doctor.

- Even the world's best doctors are no good to you if you can't get to talk to them or get an appointment in a reasonable amount of time.

4

FOUR EARS ARE BETTER THAN TWO—AND OTHER COMMUNICATION STRATEGIES

How can others help when I'm the one who is ill?

Why should I take someone to the doctor with me?

Who should go with me?

Can I bring more than one person?

Can I really use a tape recorder?

It's My Health, It's My Problem

I believe this statement is one of the great fallacies in personal health care. For those who believe it, it is also the source of great and unnecessary isolation and loneliness. It is true that we are all responsible for maintaining our own health, but **when health starts to break down, it is hard to go it alone**. Many people who get sick adopt the philosophy that they do not want to make their health problem someone else's burden. In reality, however, when you're sick, it does become a problem to those who care about you *because* they care about you!

Everyone responds differently to the stress of a diagnosis or treatment. Some people need some time alone to get their thoughts together—to center themselves. Others immediately need to be with people who care about them—people they can talk to about the situation. Many people, when faced with a serious or life-threatening illness, tend to put up a barricade as if they are in a medieval fortress surrounded by a moat. They pull up the drawbridge and keep everyone out. This creates an isolation that is counterproductive. It is not good for you, and it is not good for your loved ones. Even for those who initially need to gather themselves in private, continuing to go through a significant health problem alone is never the best strategy.

> Going through a significant
> health problem alone is never the
> best strategy.

- **How can others help when I'm the one who is ill?**
  There are many ways family and friends can help, if you let them. **In times of stress, you need the help and support of others.** You need a sounding board—someone to discuss your thoughts and fears with you. If you are mulling over the issue alone, you may be missing totally different perspectives on what is happening to you now and what lies ahead. You may be fixating on the worst possible outcome and ignoring the much-more-likely positive outcome.

  Don't worry about being a burden to your friends and family. People want to help and very often don't know how. Anyone you ask to listen or to go along to the doctor with you,

4

I believe, will feel complimented that you value them in this way and will be glad to help you.

If Bad News Could Be on the Way

As many people unfortunately find out, loneliness and isolation can be the worst part of an illness. Everyone has a need for human contact. When you are facing an illness, this need is accentuated. This is the time to share your concerns with your loved ones and to let them in. It may be hard to reach out, but if you just open the door, they will usually do the reaching out to you. **Don't be afraid to hug or be hugged.**

- **Why should I take someone to the doctor with me?**
  I can tell you from personal experience that one of the most meaningful and helpful things someone can do is to be with you when you are seeing a doctor, especially if there is the possibility that bad news is on the way. In chapter 1, I shared with you my experience with an unknown mass in my brain.

  LET ME TELL YOU MORE...
  Prior to my first visit to a neurosurgeon, I had followed my own advice to the letter. I had discussed my problem with my family doctor. I had seen a neurologist who agreed with my family physician that I needed to see a neurosurgeon. I had copies of all my tests to take with me. I had avoided any unnecessary delays in getting an appointment. Then my wife, Arlene, and I went to see the neurosurgeon together. To say that I was nervous is a great under-statement.

  I understood the possible implications of the diagnosis being considered as well as the risks of any surgery. My wife prudently decided that she would be the one driving us to the appointment. Given the options, I appreciated that the wait-and-see diagnosis he was giving me was good news. Nonetheless, you can not overestimate what a help my wife was. I found the visit very overwhelming. Not only was her presence a calming influence and a great emotional support, but also she heard everything he said.

Although there were many questions I needed to ask, I couldn't focus on them. My wife, however, while very concerned about what was being said, was able to stay focused far better than I. She was able to ask the questions that needed to be asked. Later, we repeatedly discussed it in great detail. She was able to remember parts and appreciate nuances that I was unsure of. My confidence in the doctor's recommendation came in part from knowing that Arlene read him the same way I did, both as a surgeon and a person. She was literally another set of ears at a time when I desperately needed them.

This story demonstrates how having someone with you can be critical to fully understanding what is taking place. Your spouse, however, is not always the best person.

FOR EXAMPLE...

A friend of mine, Ken, went to see a specialist because of some dizziness he was experiencing. His wife, a registered nurse, went along. Ted discussed his symptoms with the doctor, and the doctor reviewed the results of the tests that had been done. The doctor recommended surgery as the best way to correct the problem. The specialist then informed them that there was a risk that Ted could have a stroke during the surgery. About 10 minutes later, Joan stopped the doctor and asked him to back up a bit. She told me later that, essentially, she had not heard a thing after the word "stroke."

This stunned reaction is extremely common, and quite possibly the rule rather than the exception. **When bad news is given, especially when words like "cancer," "stroke," and "terminal" are used, all functional communication frequently stops.** The human brain can only process so much. When it is confronted with this type of threatening information, it frequently takes what I call a left turn. While the conversation is continuing straight down the road, the patient and sometimes the loved one are lost in their own thoughts of, "Oh my God, is this is really happening?"

Yes, it *is* happening, but I think it is important for you to recognize that many people have gone through, are going through, and will go through the same experience. Still, you can't get away from that feeling that it is only happening to you.

This is why, first and foremost, I believe when there is a possibility that bad or stressful news could be discussed, you need to have at least four ears listening.

4

- **Who should go with me?**

  Most often, but not always, if you are married, your spouse can play the role of listener. Don't forget, however, as we saw with my friend whose wife is a nurse, a spouse can take that left turn, too. Consider this before you go to the doctor: **Does your spouse have the emotional stamina to be your extra set of ears?** If not, you should take someone else.

- **Can I bring more than one person?**

  You may want to have an additional loved one with you or someone who can serve as a medical "translator." If you have a good friend or family member who is a doctor or nurse, this is ideal. If not, you may know someone who is relatively conversant in "medicalese" or someone who has had experience with the condition you are facing. Do not be worried about taking too many people with you to the doctor. Again, if you have a partnership with your doctor, she should be happy you are bringing along some more support. **The goal is to have someone there who can understand some of the nuances of what the doctor is saying.** Make sure that person understands her role.

> When bad news or stressful news may be discussed, you need at least four ears, and possibly more, listening.

Develop a Listening Plan

Once you choose your extra set of ears, you need to **discuss the listening plan with whoever is coming with you.** The reason for having four ears is so you can discuss what was said later and compare notes. Here are the elements key to your listening plan:

- Before your visit, take sufficient time to **discuss the purpose of the visit and the questions that you have. Write the questions down.** I suggest you write them out completely so you don't have to figure out what you meant by a few key words you jotted down.

- You probably want to ask the questions yourself, but **make sure someone else is keeping track so that all the questions get answered.** Often, many of your listed questions will get answered in the course of conversation with your doctor and as she addresses other concerns you bring up. Your listener can keep track of those and remind you of any still remaining on the list. This way you can focus fully on the conversation while someone else is taking it down for later review.

- If you forget questions on your list, whoever is with you should remind you, so you **get all your questions answered.**

- **Take additional paper along** and have someone else write down the answers to your questions as well as any additional questions that arise during the office visit. Often the doctor will say something that elicits a question you had not thought of before.

- Sometimes taking a **tape-recording device** is a very helpful strategy. As you know, verbal communication is not only in the words spoken but also the inflection and tone of the voice. This is why a tape recorder can be very helpful. Make sure your doctor is aware that you are recording the conversation if you choose this method.

• Can I really use a tape recorder?

I believe that when you are faced with a health crisis, getting the conversation on tape is perfectly rational and actually a smart thing to do. It can be especially important when your spouse or loved one, for whatever reason, can't go with you to an appointment.

Tape recorders provide an opportunity to revisit the conversation as often as possible to fully understand what was said. In addition, some people find that trying to write down everything the doctor says can be very distracting. The tape recorder solves that problem.

But—and this is important—if you want to record your office visit or a conversation with your doctor, you need to explain to the doctor why you want to do so before you turn it on. Tell her you would like to record the session for the reasons I just stated. Stress that as part of your medical partnership, you want to be sure that you understand her clearly. You also want to be clear what you are not trying to do—**you are not bringing the recorder along to trap the doctor or to use her words as promises.** You know how "bomb" jokes are no longer funny at the airports. Believe me, malpractice jokes are not funny in the doctor's office.

I think it is appropriate to then say, "I assume this is all right with you." If the doctor does object, or even if you sense a measure of discomfort on her part, discuss it further with her. You do not want her to distrust you. Ask why she objects. Usually, this can be worked out.

A GOOD EXAMPLE OF THIS IS:
I have a good friend who had been diagnosed with prostate cancer. He had to make a treatment decision: surgery to have his prostate removed or radiation therapy that involved implanted radioactive seeds and external beam radiation. We live in a community that is within easy driving distance to several excellent university hospitals. He chose to work with two of them. One is the world leader in treating prostate cancer through surgery. The other has a great deal of experience in treating this cancer with radiation.

My friend prudently scheduled consultations at both hospitals. His wife wanted to accompany him to these appointments as his second set of ears, but unfortunately, she couldn't. I volunteered to go with him, and we appropriately prepared and discussed our list of questions and concerns ahead of time. However, we also took a tape recorder.

We explained to the doctors the necessary absence of his wife, and they gladly agreed to our recording the conversation. At home, he and his wife could not only review our notes and reflections from the visit but also hear

> it all first-hand. I believe this gave her a much fuller appreciation for the complexity of the choice and allowed her to weigh in as an informed participant. It allowed her to be a more active advisor and supporter of her husband as he made this choice.

To me, this is a great example of **the kind of teamwork necessary for the best outcome.**

- My friend needed a second set of ears, and he had them.
- His second set of ears was also a doctor and could serve as a medical translator.
- We were prepared to listen, and we were also prepared with an advanced list of written questions.
- We recorded the office visits so his spouse could hear everything that went on as it exactly took place.

I do not advise that you call in advance for permission to record the meeting. It is likely the request will get vetoed by the staff person answering the phone. This is understandable because a face-to-face explanation to your doctor is the best way to establish trust in your true motivation. Once done, and you and your listener are with the doctor, keep these important things in mind:

- Do not turn on the tape recorder until you have your conversation with your doctor about why you want to use it.
- Do not be shy about stopping the conversation and asking the doctor to repeat what was said, even if you want the last 20 minutes repeated. The goal is to communicate, and that may require repetition.
- If your doctor is speaking in medical terms that you do not thoroughly understand, ask your doctor to explain what she's saying in layman's terms. Medical jargon can be confusing to anyone, so if you think you know what she means but you are not sure, get it clarified in simple English.
- At the end of the visit, recount what your doctor told you in your own words to make sure you understood what she was trying to communicate. Remember, the goal is for you to understand it!

A tape recorder is an especially important tool if you are the health advocate for someone else, such as an aging parent. In fact, for any person who has a memory problem or early dementia, it can be helpful for any appointment. If the patient has a memory problem, she could get home and not remember all of the doctor's advice and instructions. Or, she may have a different recollection of what the doctor said. The tape recorder is the perfect way to reassure someone that she is doing what the doctor wants, and it can be replayed as often as necessary.

After the Visit

It is very important to **discuss the visit with whomever went to the doctor with you right away while it is still fresh in your minds.** You may end up doing this many times, especially if your spouse was with you. As you think back on the visit, you may start to reanalyze what was said. This is why having notes is important. Frequently it is hard to absorb all that is said in the doctor's office during a critical time. This is especially true if what your doctor told you made you anxious. A better understanding of what was said often has a calming effect after the initial shock.

Don't shy away from reviewing the same question with your listener over and over. Also, do not hesitate to call the doctor to go over a point that is still unclear or to ask another question. Your questions and concerns are worth the doctor's time. It is to your credit that you are making sure you understand what was discussed.

> Make sure you thoroughly understand what is happening to you, even if it requires calling the doctor to understand a point further or to get more questions answered. Being unsure about anything adds to your anxiety, which you don't need.

Follow-Up Visits and a Medical Translator

If you and your companion feel that you do not totally comprehend everything that took place on that first visit, call the doctor's office and request a follow-up visit with the doctor to go over the information again. If you have a partnership with your doctor, the office will understand and make an appointment for you as soon as possible.

Don't be embarrassed at all about wanting a follow-up visit so you can review the conversation you had with your doctor. If the office resists or wants to make you wait several days, push through the resistance. Use the techniques I taught you in chapter 3. No matter how busy your doctor is, she should take the time to relieve any anxiety or clear up any confusion you have over what is happening to you. Delays are unacceptable in getting the care you need.

Key Take Home Messages

- If you think there may be bad news, take at least one other person to the doctor with you, not only for support but also to be a second pair of ears.

- Develop a listening plan for your office visit.

- After the visit, discuss what happened with whomever went to the doctor with you while it is still fresh in your minds.

- It is not unreasonable to tape record the visit.

- Do not hesitate to request a follow-up visit with the doctor to go over the information again.

5

URGENT VERSUS EMERGENT? YOU DECIDE

Do I have to worry about the difference?

How do I manage an urgent problem when I can't get in contact with my doctor?

What if I'm not sure?

Just How Sick Are You?

How responsive your doctor is to your needs at any given moment is dependent to a large degree on how you categorize the problem when you call the doctor's office. As your own medical advocate, you want to be sure that you get the care you need when you need it. In order to do this, you need to be able to differentiate among three levels of care. In other words, you need to be able to define how sick you think you are, and how soon you need to be seen by a doctor. Medicine recognizes three types of patient needs:

- **Routine** means you will be seen when it is convenient for you and the doctor. You will get an appointment at the next open time. Other then your annual check-up, this can include chronic problems like arthritis, follow-up visits that you are scheduling in advance, and the like.
- **Urgent** means that you need to be seen today. You have a new illness or injury that you do not feel is threatening to life or limb, but which does need prompt attention.
- **Emergent**, or an emergency, means you need to be seen now! There is a potential threat to life or limb like a heart attack, seizure, asthma attack, laceration, broken bone, and so on.

- **Do I have to worry about the difference?**
  The answer is an emphatic "Yes!" The way you describe what is wrong can sometimes be a matter of life or death. At the other extreme, if you overdramatize, it can create a problem of trust between you and your doctor. Sometimes it is hard to make the distinction, but you can learn how to understand the definitions so you can communicate effectively.

Routine Care

Routine care includes more than the physical examination and tests that are done as part of general preventive care. A sore shoulder that you finally decide to do something about after its been bothering you for 2 to 3 months is routine. Acne that you or your child has had for many months is routine. Any annoyance that has been bothering you for some time, and you are just getting around to doing something about, will be considered routine to the doctor when you call for an appointment—even if you feel you can't stand it for one more day.

Fortunately, **most of your lifetime care will fall into the category of routine.** This doesn't mean it is not important to you, it just means that whether it is done today or next week or even next month doesn't make a lot of medical difference. The key word here is "medical." There may be times when you are worried about a strange ache or symptom, and you want to be seen for it right away. Having to wait weeks to see your doctor may have no impact on your medical outcome, but that is of little comfort to you at that moment. **If waiting is making you anxious, then you want to see your doctor before the next routine appointment.** The important point is that **you do not have to be embarrassed about the fact that a symptom is making you nervous.**

If seeing the doctor is what you need to put your mind at ease, then call and say that you need to see the doctor as soon as possible. Ask the office staff to find a time that works for both of you. When you have a true urgent condition, you want to see your doctor now. If it is not urgent enough to be seen today, but you want to be seen as soon as possible, you must be willing to be inconvenienced about the time. It is part of your partnership. If you are feeling some resistance on the part of the doctor's office, you might have to use some of the more forceful tactics I recommend in chapter 3.

Urgent Care

My definition of an **urgent problem is one that needs attention today**. It can be a sudden illness that your doctor can not or will not satisfactorily diagnose and treat over the telephone. A possible strep throat infection, an acute ear infection, a twisted ankle that you think you sprained but you don't think you broke—these are the types of things your instinct tells you to call your doctor's office about right away. So, do it!

Call and say that you think you have an urgent medical problem that needs attention today. If you are told that the doctor will call you back, ask when. You need to be very clear that a call back at the end of the day will not work, as you believe you need to be seen today. If you are told that there are no appointments available, ask the doctor's office what they recommend you do. They are your medical partners. Don't let them be part of the problem; make them part of the solution. You do not have to accept that an urgent problem can wait until tomorrow unless you have personally spoken with the doctor.

If the staff tells you they have checked with the doctor, and relate his advice, you should follow it, unless it doesn't make sense to you. **If this is the case, insist again on speaking to the doctor. Be up front and say that you do not feel the doctor has the whole picture, and you still need to talk to him.** Patients sometimes feel that the staff has not spoken to the doctor at all and is just giving a standard response. If you feel this way, just come out and ask. There is no way of knowing if you are being lied to unless you speak to the doctor. In a patient-doctor partnership, however, this should not happen.

Whatever the directive is—a phone diagnosis or a trip to the doctor—make sure it takes place the same day. If the doctor speaks with you and feels confident that he can advise you on how to handle the situation until tomorrow, it is reasonable to follow his advice. If you can't get help from your doctor's office, head to a walk-in clinic or to the emergency room.

If you do get an appointment, realize that you may not be able to see your doctor. The office staff should do its best to make sure that you do, but you could end up being seen by another doctor, a nurse practitioner, or a certified physician's assistant in the practice. What counts most is that you are being seen in a timely fashion by a practice you trust.

> You don't have to accept the answer that an urgent problem can wait until tomorrow unless you have personally been told so by the doctor.

- **How do I manage an urgent problem when I can't get in contact with my doctor?**

  Medical problems don't pop up at the doctor's convenience. In fact, they usually happen (or at least it seems like they do) after office hours, at night, or on weekends and holidays.

  Getting urgent care during the night or weekend is sometimes easier, because many doctors use answering services with **advice nurses**. These are usually specially trained nurses who have a series of questions and protocols (steps to follow depending on how you answer the questions) available to assess the severity of your problem. If he interviews you and says the appropriate thing to do is to wait until morning and then call your doctor's office for an appointment that day, I think it is reasonable to follow his advice, provided you feel you can wait until morning. If your condition worsens or doesn't follow the course predicted, call the on-call nurse back.

  This is an issue of communication. **If you don't agree with the nurse's advice to wait, say you want to speak to the doctor. He will usually arrange this. If the answer is no or that the doctor is unavailable, go to the emergency room.** For instance, I don't think that you need to talk to the doctor personally at 4:00 in the morning for what appears to be a routine child's earache if a trained advice nurse has interviewed you and recommends how to deal with it until the doctor's office opens. The final decision is up to you, of course. Remember, if the condition worsens or doesn't improve, do something.

  > An urgent problem is one that needs attention today.

It's an Emergency!

Emergency care means that you **need medical attention not just today, but now!** These conditions cover a range of severity. For example, a cut that won't stop bleeding or looks big enough or deep enough that you think it might need stitches is an emergency. A possible broken bone is an emergency. Emergency conditions also include symptoms of a possible heart attack or stroke; any kind of head injury; or a loss of consciousness.

Your only thought should be: *Do I call my doctor's office for advice or do I just go directly to the nearest emergency room?* Depending on the severity of the above examples, sometimes the answer is obvious. If you call your doctor because he deals with these types of injuries in his office, he may tell you to come to his office, direct you to the hospital, or, if it sounds more serious, he may tell you to call 911.

> An emergency is when you need
> to be seen not just today, but now!

- **What if I'm not sure?**
Defining the status of a sudden medical situation is not always easy. As a responsible medical advocate, I suggest you think the worst: Start at emergent and work backward. **If the condition seems life- or limb-threatening to you, as a layperson, then treat it as an emergency**. It is much better to take a possibly unnecessary ambulance ride to the hospital than get tragically worse at home, and then be unable to get to a phone. As a caregiver, you don't want to be responsible for making the more conservative of two decisions and having it turn out wrong.

The natural instinct of many people who are making this decision about themselves is to resist the possibility that it could be an emergency. Don't do it! React as if someone in your care were in the same situation. The important thing is that you use your best judgment as a nonmedical caregiver. You are not expected to play doctor or make the judgment call of a doctor.

If you are not sure and feel you have time for a telephone call, then call your doctor. As soon as the person answers, **the first thing to say is "This is an emergency!" so you don't get put on hold before you can explain.** If you are still asked to be put you on hold, firmly answer "No!" You may even be put on hold before you have a chance to say anything. If this is the case, hang up and call right back and start talking as soon as the person picks up. Say it is an emergency and that you need to talk to the doctor *now*. If a nurse takes the call in response to your request, briefly tell him the problem, and then ask for the doctor. If you can't get through to the doctor, just hang up and call 911 or head to the nearest emergency room. If you speak with your doctor and he feels it is urgent rather than emergent, then go to his office instead. Again, in this type of situation, you may end up seeing one of the other doctors in the practice.

5

Key Take Home Messages

- Have a basic understanding of the difference among medical problems that are routine, urgent, or emergent.

- Know how to assess the seriousness of a condition until the doctor has a chance to tell you otherwise.

- Don't be shy about pushing as hard as necessary to get the care you need in the timeframe you think is necessary.

- When you're in doubt and you can't reach the doctor, go to the emergency room.

- If you feel it is an emergency, call 911 or go to the emergency room.

6

NOW I'M IN THE EMERGENCY ROOM!

Who uses the emergency room?

What will happen if I go to the ER?

Do they have to do all those tests?

Do I need to see my doctor, too?

The ER Is a Busy Place

If you enter the emergency room by the power of your own two feet, don't expect fast attention. Most patients spend an average of 3.2 hours in the emergency room, according to the most recent statistics. The exception, of course, is if you arrive as a true emergency—meaning by ambulance or in great physical distress.

Emergency rooms are busy places, mainly because the majority of people who show up do not have an emergency condition. Only 14 percent of the estimated 113.9 million people who visit the emergency room each year are sick or injured enough to be admitted to the hospital. Of this number, only 1.3 percent are admitted for a possible heart attack or sent to the Intensive Care Unit. This means that the vast majority (about 86 percent) of people who go to the emergency room will have to wait while injured and truly sick people are getting medical treatment. They also have to get in line behind the not-so-sick who arrived ahead of them. So, if you go to the emergency room for a nonemergent reason, anticipate a long wait (and take along a book).

- **Who uses the emergency room?**
  Everybody and anybody uses the emergency room. The name Emergency Room is kind of a misnomer because it isn't just for emergencies. For many people, especially those without insurance, the emergency room is essentially their doctor's office. By law, a hospital emergency room must at least do an initial evaluation of anyone who shows up with a complaint. Private-practice doctors, however, can choose not to see uninsured patients or people on Medicaid (a state/federal insurance plan for the indigent). So, many people feel the emergency room is their only recourse.

  This is unfortunate for them and for society as a whole. For them, it means long waits for relatively minor problems. For society, it means using one of our most complex and expensive resources at far below its intended level of care.

  If you believe you have a life- or limb-threatening injury, go to the emergency room—without hesitation. If you are not sure you are dealing with an emergency, you should **always err on**

the side of caution and go to the emergency room. Those times when you feel ill or have an urgent need to see a doctor, but your own doctor is unavailable, you should consider the emergency room. The same goes for when you get ill or are injured when you are out of town. Keep in mind, however, that when you go to the emergency room, and it is not a true emergency, you could spend hours waiting. And waiting.

6

If Your Doctor's Not In

One of the pluses of today's medical-care system is the urgent-care center or walk-in medical clinic. These facilities are geared to care for people who have sudden (acute) illnesses or minor injuries that don't need the full support of an emergency room. They can be found in many communities and resort towns. They are intended to treat you for things like a cold or flu when your doctor is unavailable.

If you are traveling, you might want to call your insurance company's Customer Service number to find out if a facility exists where you are. Your insurance company may even be able to arrange a doctor's office visit for you. In other words, if you don't have an emergency, avoid going to the emergency room if you can!

Some emergency rooms have an urgent-care center integrated into the facility. These combined units function by sorting the urgent from the emergency patients and sending them to the appropriate medical teams. This is good if you have an urgent problem because you most likely will be treated quicker.

As a medical advocate for yourself and your family, **you should familiarize yourself with the hospitals in your community and the emergency facilities they offer.**

> Hospital emergency rooms are heavily utilized. Some of the people there are very ill, quite possibly more ill than you, so be prepared to wait.

Checking into the ER

How you arrive at the ER is the first clue to the seriousness of your condition. **If you arrive by ambulance, the ER staff is already on alert.** You will bypass the registration desk and be taken to the treatment area. (If someone is with you, however, they may be asked to sign you in). The emergency-room doctor and/or nurse will do an initial evaluation on you as rapidly as possible and decide how soon you need more in-depth assessment and treatment. **Fast attention is one of the advantages of calling an ambulance when you have a true emergency.** The other advantage is that the emergency medical technicians will assess you and begin providing care while transporting you to the hospital.

In cases other than a true emergency, you will be registered at the intake desk, and then asked to go to the waiting room. A triage nurse (someone specially trained to make a fast evaluation) will see you, and if she feels you need immediate attention, she will facilitate your rapid transfer to the treatment area.

Communicate honestly with the triage nurse. **If you believe you have an emergency condition, say so.** If she doesn't agree and you are asked to wait and your condition begins to deteriorate, go back to the registration desk and reinforce the emergent nature of your problem. Because of the large number of patients who use the emergency room for nonemergent conditions, sometimes the emergency-room staff at first under-estimates the severity of a patient's condition. You need to be your own advocate in this setting. If you need care immediately, make sure they know it!

- **What will happen if I go to the ER?**
  Once you are in the treatment area, a thorough evaluation will be performed. This will begin with an appropriate medical history and physical to understand why you are there and how ill you are. If you need **testing** such as laboratory tests or x-rays, they will be done. If you need specialized x-rays or tests, or if you need the care of a specialist, you may need to wait longer for those people to arrive. In other words, **if you are sick and need treatment that is beyond the scope of what ER personnel**

typically do, you could be in for a long wait. No matter how sick you are, expect some prolonged waiting periods during your visit to the ER.

- **Do they have to do all those tests?**

The emergency team knows very little or nothing about you and your medical background. In order to treat you properly, the ER doctor may need to order a broad range of tests all at once to sort out your symptoms as quickly as possible and to find out what is happening. On the other hand, if you were in your own doctor's office, she would have both her past personal knowledge of your care and history as well as the results from any prior tests. She likely would need to do far less testing to get the same results. This is another thing that adds to the expense of running an emergency room.

- **Do I need to see my doctor, too?**

If the ER solves your problem, you don't have to see your doctor, but you do need to **let your doctor know that you were there.** You should ask the **ER to send a copy of the records and test results to your doctor. Do not depend on the hospital to do this on its own.** It is also important that you follow the instructions the ER gives you, unless your doctor informs you otherwise.

For instance, the ER may instruct you to come back to the ER for some follow-up care, which your doctor feels she can provide better in her office. Or, the ER physician might also refer you to a specialist for follow-up. Whatever the outcome of your visit to the ER, you should **check with your doctor first to see if she agrees that more attention is required.** She may have an alternative suggestion. Talk to her about it and then proceed to get the care you need.

A Word to the Wise

If you are sick enough to go to the ER, this means that you should not go alone. **Have someone drive you and stay with you until you are sent home or get a diagnosis.** Even if you are capable of driving yourself to the ER, you may need someone to drive you home, because the treatment may involve medications or procedures that will limit your ability to safely drive yourself home. If your condition is serious, having someone with you is very important because she can also serve as your **additional pair of ears to help you better understand what the doctors are telling you.**

Communication in the ER is often very difficult not only because you are sick but also because of the busy environment of the emergency room.

> Have someone go to the ER
> with you!

Key Take Home Messages

- Lots of people use the emergency room whether they are seriously ill or not, so take a book and expect to wait.

- Because the ER is unfamiliar with your medical condition, you may have to go through otherwise unnecessary tests.

- When in doubt, go to the emergency room.

- Let your doctor know you were there and have the ER send a copy of the records to your doctor.

- Take someone with you to the ER!

TESTS AND OTHER PROCEDURES

If the doctor orders a test, does it mean it is necessary?

Can I say no?

Is there a different test I can take?

Will the test be covered by my insurance?

The Age of Medical Testing

Testing is playing an ever-increasing role in medical evaluations. Despite insurance companies clamoring for doctors to do less testing to save money, the trend over recent years is going in the opposite direction. I believe there are a number of forces driving this trend.

Advances in medical science means advances in testing methods. There are more sophisticated testing mechanisms that allow doctors to discover and diagnose problems faster— meaning life-threatening diseases can be found earlier and, thus lives are saved. Also, new uses of existing testing methods are being found. This is true for both laboratory testing, such as blood tests, and for imaging testing, such as x-rays, CT scans, and MRI studies. Our ability to "see" what is going on in the body appears to be more and more miraculous with each passing year.

I also believe that the rising number of malpractice lawsuits has created a climate in which physicians are motivated both by their desire to get the best treatment for their patients and by the perceived need to have a paper trail proving that no stone was left unturned. **Rather than just do the tests they feel are most appropriate, many physicians are practicing "defensive medicine"** and doing tests that they believe are only remotely useful, all in order to avoid any charges that they were not thorough enough. This is unfortunate, and it does not serve the patient, or society as a whole, very well.

As a result, more than 10 billion laboratory tests and 500 million imaging procedures are being performed in the United States annually, according to recent statistics. This comes to about 35 lab tests and two imaging exams for every person in the country. That's a lot of testing!

> Nowadays, tests are done extremely frequently. Managing your health care includes managing testing. Overtesting, like undertesting, can be harmful.

- **If the doctor orders a test, does it mean it is necessary?**

  Just because a test is ordered by your doctor does not mean it is necessary. One of the things you, as your own medical advocate, want to understand when any test or procedure is proposed is why. It is completely within your right and most certainly within your best interest to ask:

  - What impact will this test have on the management of my illness?
  - What are the benefits and risks?
  - Is this the proper time in my care for this test?

  7

  For every test, there should be an expected benefit from the information learned. That goes for anything from a blood cholesterol test to a heart catheterization that looks for blockage in arteries leading to your heart. A test is only necessary if it will aid in your care, so you need to know how the information will affect your diagnosis or treatment. If it won't affect your treatment, why do it? This even includes tests that are considered health-screening tests: cholesterol tests, blood sugar tests, mammograms, and so on. If your doctor is ordering a screening test, he should be comfortable explaining how the test will allow him to alter your care if it reveals any abnormality.

  > FOR EXAMPLE . . .
  > After the radiologist saw my first MRI, which is generally the best test for looking at the structure of the brain, he recommended a CT scan of my brain as well. I asked why, since both are imaging studies. He said that sometimes harmless calcifications can create suspicious findings on an MRI. Only a CT scan would show if this was the case. Essentially, it would make a major difference in my diagnosis and treatment. I had the test, and a significant calcification was there. This supported the watch-and-wait approach we were taking.

  Your doctor may say the test will make him feel better about the treatment plan. Ask him what he means. Doctors often say this because they have some degree of uncertainty and want further evidence that they are on the right track. If this is the case, he should be able to clarify this for you. If he is only ordering tests to "cover all the bases," and there is no reasonable likelihood the tests will help in your care, this is not good enough! Remember, the goal is to make *you* feel better, not the doctor.

This is not to say that tests are a waste of time. Tests are a valuable part of medical diagnosis and treatment. The important point is that they should be done only if the results will affect the diagnosis or treatment. The reason to not do a test has nothing to do with helping the insurance company save money. The reason is because **every test carries a risk.**

> A test should affect your
> diagnosis and treatment, or else
> it isn't necessary.

There Are Risks in Everything

There is always some risk involved both in the performance and in knowing the results of a test. The risk in the performance may be fairly minimal, like pain or bruising from having blood drawn. More complex procedures carry greater risks. For example, the risks associated with heart catheterization, a procedure in which x-ray dye is injected into the arteries to find out if blood is flowing freely into the heart, include injury to the arteries of your heart or an allergic reaction to the dye.

But there are risks besides physical injury. The results can include information that makes the doctor suspect some other unrelated condition may exist, which means he will want to do more tests. Sure, this can lead to the discovery of a new and unsuspected problem, but more often chasing "accidental" findings causes unnecessary additional testing that ultimately leads nowhere.

AN EXAMPLE...
I have a friend, Elizabeth, who fell and had injured her chest

wall. She went to the emergency room where she got an x-ray of her ribs. It did not show any fractures. Well-aligned rib fractures may not show up on the initial x-ray. In fact, it can take about 10 days to show as the changes of healing appear. Elizabeth continued to have pain, which was consistent with rib fractures. However, when she told her doctors of the continuing pain, they recommended a chest CT scan before the 10 days were up. The scan found three questionable changes in her chest wall and upper abdomen, which resulted in her having multiple other tests, including more CT scans. All the "changes" turned out to be insignificant. In the meantime, when she got the 10-day rib x-ray, she found out she had two broken ribs. All the additional testing was unnecessary.

7

It is tempting to say, "So what, it's better to be safe than sorry!" However, the key question that you need to remember to ask is, *How likely is it that this test will produce results that will help manage my illness?* In my friend's situation, a few days' wait would have resolved her concerns without additional inconvenience, expense, and exposure to radiation.

You Can Quantify the Risks

Your doctor should be able to tell you the benefits and risks of a test. For most tests with significant risk, such as those that use cardiac catheterization or other studies that use x-ray dye, **these risks have been quantified, and your doctor can tell you what percent of patients have complications.** Often, the more invasive the test, the more data is available. Don't be afraid to ask your doctor for these numbers. Your doctor may never have personally seen some of the uncommon complications, but they may still happen often enough for you not to want the test. How much risk you take should be determined by how much benefit the test offers.

FOR INSTANCE. . .
A relative, Jim, who was having pain in his leg, spoke with

me after being referred by his neurologist for a nerve biopsy. This is a procedure in which a small portion of a nerve is surgically removed, then tested for abnormalities under the microscope. Although we think of biopsies usually with cancer, they can be done for a variety of reasons. The neurosurgeon who would be performing the test told Jim that he could end up with chronic nerve pain as a result of the biopsy.

I suggested that he go back to the neurosurgeon and ask some more questions before he agreed to have the test. A key question to ask was *what percentage of patients have chronic pain after biopsy?* I encouraged him to inquire about medical studies on nerve biopsies. Physicians should be able to produce this information easily. This led to a very detailed conversation with the neurosurgeon, and allowed Jim to understand the benefits and risks of the procedure.

The bottom line was that Jim found out that there was a low probability of finding anything on the biopsy. Further, treatment had already begun on the condition the doctor was looking for. He declined to have the nerve biopsy!

> The more specific questions
> you ask about risks and benefits,
> the better you can decide what
> is right for you!

- **Can I say no?**
  Yes! You are a partner in your medical care. Whether the suggestion for a medical test comes from you primary-care physician or a specialist, **you have the right to refuse the test**. You should get your doctor's opinion as to why he wants you to have the test. I would strongly suggest that you discuss your reasons for wanting to reject the test with your doctor. He frequently will be able to resolve your concerns. If in the end you don't want it, you still have the right to say no.

- **Is there a different test I can take?**

  Sometimes your doctor will propose a test that you are uncomfortable with. For instance, your doctor wants you to get an MRI of your brain, but the thought of being surrounded by the "doughnut" of the MRI machine makes you nervous. Ask about alternatives. Your doctor may suggest some anti-anxiety medicine for you to take during the exam. He might suggest doing the test at a facility that offers open-air MRIs, where the patient is not enclosed by MRI apparatus. Though open MRIs often don't give quite as sharp an image as the closed MRIs, they are a great alternative for some patients. The doctor might even suggest some other way to get information on your condition without requiring a MRI. You won't know if you don't ask! Remember, your doctor is making his first recommendation to you. It is very possible that he has two or three ways to solve the problem. Doctors do not always offer you a choice unless you ask.

  > Before agreeing to a test, ask about the alternatives.

- **Will the test be covered by my insurance?**

  Whether the test is covered, of course, depends on your insurance, and it is something you should find out ahead of time. Your doctor can have the office check for you. For some insurance plans, there are only certain providers and certain facilities that are included in the insurance plan's network. Asking in advance of the test is important. In addition, some policies may require that you pay a co-pay or some percentage of the cost of a given test.

  Tests are not cheap. For example, a routine red and white blood cell count in my community costs about $65, while the charge for a complete MRI of the brain costs about $2,000. Most insurance companies do not pay the list price for the tests. However, if you get testing done and have to pay for it out of pocket, you have to pay the list price. If one test leads to another, as demonstrated in the case of my friend with the broken ribs, your out-of-pocket costs can add up in a hurry. A necessary cost if it saves your health, but a waste of money (the insurance company's too!) if the test will not change the diagnosis or treatment.

If you have any questions about who pays the costs, look in your insurance benefit booklet or call your insurance company. Just because it is listed as not covered doesn't mean that you can't get your insurance company to pay for it. (For strategies on getting your insurance company to pay for procedures not covered, see chapter 24).

Key Take Home Messages

- Ask why your doctor is proposing a test, and if it is necessary. Find out how it will change your diagnosis or treatment.

- Know the benefits and risks of any medical test you are taking.

- Don't be shy about asking about alternatives.

- Check beforehand if the test is covered by your insurance at the facility you plan to use.

- If the test is not covered, work with your insurance company to get it covered.

8

FOLLOW-UP—
IT'S UP TO YOU

When will I get my results?

How should I get the results?

I'm worried — can I get my results sooner?

What if the results are a surprise?

Which result should I trust?

What happens when a different test changes
my diagnosis?

A Critical Part of Your Care

Whether you've had a simple blood test or major surgery, having a clear understanding of the follow-up plan, then making sure it is followed, is one of the most critical parts of ensuring that you are receiving the best medical care. From my experience managing a medical practice, I believe that **this is the responsibility of both the doctor and the patient.** But as your own medical advocate, consider it your own responsibility. It is far too important to you to leave it totally up to the doctor. Don't forget, it is your health at stake!

Test Results

The term follow-up can cover a vast array of medical situations but the most common is finding out the results of tests you've had done. I would encourage you to not accept the approach that no news is good news. The truth is: No news is no news! You want to hear back from your doctor on the results. Why? Because **no news can mean that the results of the test never made it back to your doctor**. Or it can mean that the results came back, but someone in the office filed it away before you were ever contacted.

Though it is rare, laboratories do lose blood tests or have a problem transmitting results to a doctor, meaning they may never show up. Though you might assume the doctor's office is watching and waiting for your tests to arrive, things can slip through the cracks of a medical practice just like anywhere else. It is up to you to make sure this doesn't happen.

- **When will I get my results?**
  It is important for you to ask at the time you are getting the test done when you can expect the results. Get a clear understanding of when and how you should get the results. Write the date down on your calendar so if you haven't heard, you can call your doctor. **Don't agree to a plan in which she will only contact you if the results are not what she expects.**

No news is no news! If you haven't heard the results of your test when you expected to, call your doctor and ask about the results.

• How should I get the results?

How you get the results depends on the kind of test you are having and why you are having it. If you and your physician think you are dealing with a minor problem, then a telephone call or a letter may work well for communicating the results. If you have a complex or serious illness, or if you expect that you'll want to talk to your physician about the test results, then you may want to make an appointment to review the results, so the two of you can plan the next phase of your medical care at that time.

8

Sometimes the doctor may get the results and feel she needs to discuss them with you personally. Then, even if the original plan was to call you or write to you, she may have her office call you and ask you to come in for an appointment. The important thing is to **pick a communication approach that lets you fully understand the results of the test** and where you go from there.

• I'm worried—can I get my results sooner?

How soon you should get the results back depends on a number of variables.

THIS IS ONE OF THEM...

I have a friend, Linda, who has had a number of mammo-grams over the years. Unfortunately, she has breasts that are very difficult to evaluate on both a mammography and physical examination. Because of this, she frequently gets called back for additional x-ray views or ultrasound examinations to help in the diagnosis. As you can imagine, with each succeeding examination, Linda has gotten more and more concerned about the results. The mammography office she goes to has a policy to mail a letter with the results and follow-up recommendations to the patient. Waiting for this letter has become more and more stressful to her.

We talked about this, and I helped her arrange for a

same-day reading of the results to be relayed to her by telephone, also on the same day. I also suggested that she arrange her appointments when the radiologist whom she trusts the most is in the office. This provides her quick feedback and consistent communication of the results.

The lesson in this story is that sometimes **the timing of getting the results can be almost as important to your sense of well-being as the results.** For many people, this is not an issue, but if it is for you, you should work with your doctor to develop a strategy that gets you prompt results within hours, not days, of when the data is available.

- **What if the results are a surprise?**

For most tests, you and your doctor usually will have a general expectation of the results. You are not absolutely certain, of course, or else you wouldn't need the test. If the results vary somewhat from what was expected (or hoped for), then that variation should guide future care. Sometimes, however, the results are far from expected. This could mean one of two things: The results are right, in which case you and your doctor will talk about the next step, or the results are wrong. But how are you to know? I suggest you talk about any "surprise results" with your doctor. If it is a simple test, like a blood test, I recommend **you repeat the test**.

A FRIEND OF MINE HAD SUCH A PROBLEM...
She got the results of her cholesterol reading, which was a routine part of her annual physical. The laboratory reported her total cholesterol was 289, high by any measure. Her last test a year earlier showed her total cholesterol was only 189, which was quite good. The new test indicated that she went from a cholesterol level considered better than average to one that is considered significantly at risk. Her doctor discussed with her options to lower her cholesterol with diet and/or medication. Before proceeding with any change, however, they decided to repeat the test. The repeat test was below 200 and essentially unchanged from one year ago.

The assumption was that the lab test in conflict with all the other medical findings was abnormal and due to some type of laboratory error. Deciding how soon to do the next follow-up test is part of the art of medicine.

Although I believe great care is taken to ensure that tests are done properly and results are issued to the correct patient, **errors do occur.** If as discussed, you have had normal cholesterol readings for many years, and then a test puts you far above where you have always been, do not panic. The next logical step is to ask your doctor if there is any medical reason she knows that would account for this.

Unless there is a good explanation, request that the test be repeated now—not 3 to 6 months from now. You want to repeat the test promptly, because if the results are correct, you need to institute some treatment plan. However, you don't want to start a treatment program on the basis of a lab result that does not make sense in view of your total medical evaluation.

> If the result of a test doesn't make sense or is a surprise, insist that the test be repeated—now!

- **Which result should I trust?**

If you repeat a test and the result varies greatly from the first test, which do you trust? Did the laboratory make a mistake on the first test or the repeat test? Don't delude yourself into assuming the value you want must be the correct one. On the other hand, you don't want to take a third test. In my experience as a radiologist, I believe the answer lies in the medical context of the result. By this I mean **the result that makes the most sense in view of your medical history.** Discuss this with your doctor and ask questions so you can leave feeling comfortable with this judgment. This helps you get to the correct diagnosis in the shortest time.

FOR INSTANCE...
I know someone with hepatitis C, an often-incurable virus infection of the liver that had been inactive for some time. One of her routine blood tests revealed that she had

elevated liver enzymes, an indication that the condition was active. However, elevated liver enzymes can indicate other things as well, so her doctor ordered a series of blood tests, many of which were interpreted as abnormal. Grave's disease, a condition involving an overactive thyroid, was considered likely.

She was referred to an endocrinologist for further evaluation and testing. The endocrinologist concluded the abnormal thyroid tests were not correct and that my friend did not have Grave's disease. So, she was sent back to her doctor, who did additional testing for changes in her hepatitis. The original liver test was repeated "just to be sure." When the evaluation was finished, the doctors found that her hepatitis C had become active and the necessary treatment was begun.

This story again shows how evaluating a test in the context of the patient's current state of health and other test results can help a doctor decide the accuracy of the findings. Had this woman's doctors started to treat her for a possible thyroid condition after her first blood test, her recurrent liver problem would have gone untreated.

> Your medical tests need to be evaluated in the context of your current state of health and your medical history.

- **What happens when a different test changes my diagnosis?**

A diagnosis can change when a doctor or even a team of doctors are not certain what is wrong with a patient. This can cause a distressing string of conflicting diagnoses and/or treatment plans.

A PERFECT EXAMPLE OF THIS IS MY OWN EXPERIENCE...

As I discussed earlier, I had a series of MRIs of my head and am now being cared for at one of the country's premier university hospitals. Before I see my neurosurgeon, I have

9

THERE IS MORE THAN ONE WAY TO SKIN A CAT

What treatment is out there that is not being proposed and why?

What about the Internet?

Know Your Options

There is no way around it. During a lifetime, there are many times a body requires repair and conditioning. When it does, your doctor will recommend a proposed course of treatment.

Even if you have the best relationship with your doctor that you feel you could possibly have—even if you trust him implicitly—you should not merely nod and say "okay." There are questions you want to ask before you agree to anything. First, **you want to be sure that you understand what is being suggested.** Related to this, **you want to understand why he has chosen this course of treatment instead of an alternative.** You also want to **know why he is suggesting this now instead of having done it sooner or waiting until later.**

A GOOD EXAMPLE OF THIS IS...

My friend, Greg, was seeing an orthopedic surgeon because of degenerative changes in his hip from osteoarthritis. The surgeon had been working with him to help manage the pain of the condition. Finally, he suggested that my friend have a total hip replacement. The surgeon explained that he thought my friend had achieved as much benefit as he could expect from his medications and nonsurgical care. He also said that he did not think there was anything to be gained from physical therapy.

In terms of the timing, the surgeon said that when the hip hurt more than the thought of surgery, the surgery should be scheduled. The operation the surgeon recommended was the standard total hip replacement widely performed at the time.

Greg told me about his upcoming surgery and asked me what I thought. I told him about an article I had recently read discussing a new technique that involved a much smaller incision and a much faster healing time. I suggested he ask his doctor about this option before he proceeded with the standard surgery. He did.

His surgeon said he was aware of the procedure, but there were only a very few medical centers in the country performing it. He also said he had no experience with the new technique and could not do it. Fortunately, we live close to a major medical school and teaching hospital. We called the school and other major medical centers in our area to find out if they performed the procedure Greg was interested in. He found a doctor who does the procedure and made an appointment to see him.

The new surgeon discussed the pros and cons of the procedure in general and specifically in regard to my friend's case. Greg has a somewhat complex medical history, which he discussed with the surgeon, that made this less-invasive surgical approach a real advantage to him. He subsequently had the less-invasive surgery and a more rapid recovery than was expected with the standard approach. Today, he is doing just fine.

9

This story is significant because it is an example of how **being aware of as many options as possible can lead to the best course of action for you.** Keep in mind, however, that the newest approach may be great for one person, but it might not be the best for you. For instance, the small-incision hip surgery was great for my friend who is normal weight. If he had been obese, this approach might not have been an option. The thickness of the tissue around his hip might have precluded this approach. Another friend could not have the small-incision surgery because her hip disease was more complex. She benefited from the surgeon having the greater visibility that the standard incision allows.

> Investigate all your options before committing to a course of treatment. Choose the one that is best for you.

The State of the Art

Frequently in medicine there is a consensus reached among doctors as to what is considered the "state-of-the-art" approach for some conditions. In my experience as both a physician and as a medical administrator, **this term refers to the best practice**

that is widely available. There is agreement that it is the very best *proven* approach. It is not referring to as-yet-unproven and experimental approaches.

If state-of-the-art treatment is something you want to explore—and you should—it may mean bringing another doctor into your fold—what we call a sub-specialist.

FOR INSTANCE...

I know an excellent mammographer (radiologist who specializes in breast imaging), Ruth, who, unfortunately, was diagnosed with breast cancer herself. She chose a surgeon from a regional facility dedicated to the treatment of breast disease. I asked her how she made her choice. She told me that she personally knew the surgeon and felt comfortable with her, and that the surgeon did a procedure call sentinel lymph node biopsy as part of the surgery.

This approach was the state-of-the-art at the time. It involves injecting a small amount of radioactive material into the breast tumor prior to surgery, which allows the surgeon to identify the best probable lymph nodes to biopsy to look for evidence of spread of the tumor. The procedure was done, and a microscopic tumor was found. This state-of the art approach allowed for more precise diagnosis and, therefore, more precise treatment of my friend.

> If there is a state-of-the-art approach for your illness, you want to discuss it as part of your treatment choices.

RECENTLY I RECEIVED A CALL FROM ANOTHER FRIEND...

She had just had a mammogram that showed some suspicious new calcifications. Sometimes a breast tumor can be seen on a mammogram as only abnormal calcifications without a tumor mass being visible. The radiologist told her that there was a low probability that they were malignant, but that he couldn't be sure without some form of biopsy. She was scheduled for a stereotaxic needle biopsy (a state-of-the-art approach using an x-ray-guided needle to biopsy areas of possible breast cancer).

Prior to the needle biopsy, she was scheduled for a surgical consultation. She asked me what questions she should ask the surgeon. She understood that this was only a consultation, because, if the biopsy was negative, no surgery would be needed. I suggested that in addition to the usual questions, she should ask the surgeon what he thought the probability was that it was cancer. I also told her to ask how many breast surgeries he performed each year, and if he used a radioactive tracer to facilitate a sentinel lymph node biopsy—the procedure described in the previous story. If that was part of his general approach, that was great. If not, she should discuss with him why not and consider finding a surgeon who was using this approach. I suggested that if she wanted to look for another surgeon, she could ask her mammographer, who worked with breast surgeons on a daily basis.

9

The point of this story is that you want to be aware of the state-of-the-art treatment and use it if it is appropriate for you. If such an option exists and your doctor doesn't do it, the earlier you know, the earlier you can consider whether you need to change physicians or **add an additional physician to your health-care team.**

This last concept is an important one. Sometimes, it may be best not to change your whole care team, but just add an additional member who brings a specific expertise you want. This is particularly helpful when you have an already trusting relationship with the doctors caring for you.

The Pros and Cons of Each

It is important to keep in mind that just because there is a new treatment available does not mean it is necessarily the best choice for you. This could be a reason why your doctor doesn't even raise the issue. **You do, however, have the right to explore all the options, but you must also realize that there are pros and cons to everything.**

One of the major cons to any new procedure is that it is new: Only a limited number have actually been performed at the time it is first discussed in the medical literature. Also, there is usually an absence of long-term follow-up data available. Common post-operative problems hopefully will have been already discovered, but uncommon and rare problems often have not. A procedure has to be done a lot of times to encounter all the uncommon and rare events. The obvious pro to a new procedure is that it often is a significant improvement over the old way of doing the surgery.

> Explore the alternatives and understand that there are pros and cons to everything.

Another pick-and-choose scenario is when there is more than one established method of treatment. There will be pros and cons to each, and you must choose among them. This dilemma is frequently encountered by women with breast cancer. Sometimes the best approach seems clear to all. In other cases, however, the pros and cons of each must be carefully evaluated to reach a decision that is right for the individual.

Realize that evaluating pros and cons can be difficult, and it will always produce different decisions by different people. This is because the decisions are often based on your value system. Let's stay with our example of breast cancer treatment. For some women, having the breast removed offers the maximum possibility of a cure and this is the highest priority.

For others, issues of body image are paramount and, to these women, a slightly lower chance of a cure may be acceptable to preserve the best body appearance. Options like radiation, chemotherapy, and surgery may be more or less preferable depending on what you have seen and heard about the effects from people you know.

For example, if your friend had a particularly stormy experience with radiation therapy, you might want to avoid radiation therapy for yourself. You need to evaluate the options carefully, weighing your values and concerns. Discussing them in detail with your physician is an important conversation. This is also an important discussion to have with your loved ones and/or friends.

- **What treatment is out there that is not being proposed and why?**

> IMAGINE...
>
> You enter your surgeon's office and he lays out three possibilities. The first he says he can do but does not recommend it, and he tells you why. The second he can also do, the risks are less than 2 percent, and you'd probably fare well. But he says there is another newer approach that is very promising and that you are an excellent candidate. He writes you a referral and says that you are welcome to come back if you decide it is not for you.

This is a wonderful scenario, but medical consultations often do not proceed this way. This is not to say that your doctor means to do you a disservice. **Your doctor's job is to make a recommendation on his best judgment, and in many doctors' minds, that is a judgment based on his own experience and capabilities.** However, there are a variety of reasons your doctor may not have offered you all the options, and they include:

- Your doctor may not be aware of all the options.
- Your doctor may have considered other options, and is giving you his best recommendation.
- Your doctor may know certain options require travel to a distant health-care facility, and he knows some patients don't want to do this.
- Your doctor may be concerned that your insurance will not cover certain options.
- Your doctor may feel that new options need more study before they are offered to patients in general.
- Your doctor may think you want him to care for you and is only giving you options he can provide.
- Your doctor may not want to lose you as a patient.

Therefore, part of being your own patient advocate is **exploring the options with your doctor prior to committing to a plan of treatment.** Even if you and your doctor have a good relationship, you should always ask: *What are all my options?* Also ask him why he is recommending one and is not recommending another.

Even if your physician already has evaluated all the available options and offered his best recommendation, you want to discuss why he chose that course of treatment. Don't forget, you may have a different opinion! As in my friend's hip surgery, there may be an alternative that your doctor doesn't recommend that is better for you. No matter why your doctor chooses his recommendation, **you want to be part of deciding what is best for you.**

I believe that you will often agree with your doctor's recommendation once you have heard the pros and cons of all your options — but not always. Medical decisions about your health are too important to you to not ask this question.

> You want to know what other options exist before you commit to a plan.

• What about the Internet?

Even after you've heard your doctor out, you may feel you want to do a little research on your own before making a decision. One way is to discuss it with friends you may have in a health-care profession, who may be able to steer you to other doctors or know about other options. Or, discuss it with people you know and trust who have been through a similar experience or know someone who has been through it. However, be very cautious about taking secondhand advice. Things often can be lost or misinterpreted in translation. If information is being passed to you from a third party, make the effort to speak directly to this person.

An alternative source of information, of course, is the Internet. I discuss the pros and cons of this approach in chapter 17, but for now I will say that you have to be very careful about the source of what you are reading.

Whatever information you discover on your own, it is in your best interest to take the information to your doctor for an informed discussion. Your doctor most likely will have insights that will be helpful to you in making your decision.

Your Insurance Company Is Not the Boss!

It is possible that an option won't be presented to you because your doctor believes that your insurance doesn't routinely cover it. **You need to separate the best medical decision from what your insurance will cover.** Push your doctor to discuss all the medical options first. If your preferred approach is a problem for your insurance policy, then you should begin working on your insurance company. The approaches you can take to this type of insurance problem are discussed in chapter 24. The bottom line is that you do not have to take no for an answer!

9

Key Take Home Messages

- Make sure you thoroughly understand the treatment your doctor is suggesting.

- Tell your doctor you want to hear about all options, including the ones he can't perform.

- Get the pros and cons for all your options.

- Find out if there is a state-of-the-art approach to your problem and discuss it with your doctor.

- Separate the best medical decision from what your insurance will cover.

- The final choice is yours.

10

SECOND OPINIONS—HOW TO MAKE THE CALL

Must I get a second opinion?

Whom should I go to for a second opinion?

Should I get the second opinion from a doctor in a different specialty?

How do I make an appointment for a second opinion?

If the second opinion disagrees with my doctor's opinion, what should I do?

Can I use the second-opinion doctor as an ongoing resource?

Should I get a third or fourth opinion?

When in Doubt

First, let me say this: There is nothing wrong with getting a second opinion. In fact, there are a lot of things right about getting a second opinion. **A second opinion is probably a good idea if:**

- A diagnosis comes at you totally out of the blue.
- You are told that you have some rare or unusual disease— even if it is not life-threatening.
- There are several ways to treat your problem and you are not convinced that the one your doctor is recommending is the one you want.

- **Must I get a second opinion?**
  You do not have to get a second opinion. Can you get a second opinion? The answer to this is, yes—it is always your call. When to know if you should get one is the crux of the matter.

  There are times when a second opinion will be of no help to you. For instance, you have a straightforward medical problem, such as a hernia, and you and your doctor have discussed your options. You have agreed on an approach that she can do. You feel comfortable with the decision. This is a common situation, particularly for less-complicated or non-life-threatening conditions.

  However, what if you are given a very serious diagnosis and told there will be a bad outcome no matter what is done?

> FOR INSTANCE...
> Lynn, an ophthalmologist I know, had a rule that whenever she made a diagnosis that meant a patient would ultimately go blind, she told the patient to get a second opinion at one of the two nearby university medical centers. It was not that she lacked confidence, and to my knowledge, there was never a case in which the university doctor came up with a significantly different diagnosis or treatment plan. It's just that she thought, considering the diagnosis, that the patient deserved a second opinion from a consulting specialist to make sure every option had been considered.

No doctor is infallible, and a second opinion can be good reassurance to a patient that all options are being explored. A competent physician should not be threatened by one.

Second opinions, however, are not for every patient. No matter what the circumstances, there are some people who will not want one, and that is fine, too. Some patients feel more comfortable and think they will do better if they follow the advice of their doctor. For them, the need to feel the confidence in their own doctor is more important than any reassurance they might gain from consulting with another specialist. I believe that feeling good about the care you are receiving is a critical part of your care and will impact on your sense of health and well-being.

> A second opinion can be good reassurance that all opinions are being explored, but some patients may be more comfortable not getting one.

10

• **Whom should I go to for a second opinion?**
I believe that, most often, the way to find the best person to give a second opinion is to **discuss it with your doctor and ask for a recommendation.** If you have a good relationship with your doctor, she will not take it as an insult. If she seems threatened or insulted, don't ignore that. Tell her that you are not challenging the value of the care she is providing you. You are fulfilling your part of the partnership by thoroughly examining all your options and making sure you are informed.

A somewhat controversial concern is whether you can get a valid second opinion from a doctor who is in the same medical practice as your doctor. I personally believe you can, but I know many people are uncomfortable doing so. These patients have a concern that physicians who work together may go out of their way to be supportive of each other. Because physicians are partners does not mean, to me, that they will tell you exactly the same thing. However, if you are concerned about this, it is perfectly all right to see a doctor from a different medical practice.

Another option is to go to a doctor in your community who is particularly respected in her field. **If there is a medical school nearby, going to one of the faculty that specializes in your condition** is another excellent source.

Asking for a second opinion does not mean you are shopping for a new physician. Let your doctor know this. You should be up front with your doctor and say that you will be back to see her to discuss the second opinion. In fact, one of the big advantages of discussing your plans for a second opinion with your doctor is that her office can be prepared to forward all your tests and other findings to the second physician in advance of your appointment. Be clear when you are making that appointment that you are looking for a second opinion and will be taking it back to your own doctor.

- **Should I get the second opinion from a doctor in a different specialty?**

  If there is more than one specialty that manages your condition, it is often a good idea to choose a doctor from another specialty for your second opinion. For example, in chapter 4, I told the story of a friend who had prostate cancer. The disease was diagnosed by an urologist, who does surgery to remove the prostate in cancer patients. But the disease can also be treated through radiation therapy, so my friend went to a radiation oncologist (a radiation therapy specialist) for his second opinion.

  The problem with seeing specialists with different techniques is that the specialist usually believes her approach is the best for the patient. After all, if they didn't believe that, why would they have chosen that specialty? However, part of your evaluation of any proposed medical treatment is to understand the benefits and success rates and the risks and complications of any approach. By understanding these, you will be amazed how easy some decisions become.

  > Sometimes you can get the full scope of options only if you talk to physicians in more than one specialty.

What It Is Not

A second opinion does not mean that you will have to go through all the testing and examinations that resulted in your original diagnosis all over again. The second-opinion doctor will base her opinion on the same results your treating doctor used. This is why you must **be sure to take all your records, tests, and other consultation reports with you or have them forwarded to the doctor prior to your appointment.** Though the doctor will not repeat the testing, she may want to repeat key parts of the physical examination.

FOR INSTANCE. . .

One of my daughters, Amy, is a singer and was having vocal cord problems. She went to a university hospital for a second opinion. She took along all of her prior medical records and tests. The new doctor still wanted to take a look at her vocal cords himself, and he also asked many questions about her symptoms. She did not have to repeat an extensive work-up, however, because she had the records with her. She got her second opinion and recommendation and took the information back to her treating physician.

10

A second opinion should not mean that you are shopping for another doctor.

- **How do I make an appointment for a second opinion?**
  The best approach for a second opinion is to do it very openly. If you are in a managed-care health plan, you probably will need to ask your primary-care physician for a referral for the second opinion. Then, you will have to call the second specialist's office for an appointment for a second opinion. Remember, this is a common practice, so you don't have to feel awkward about it.

- **If the second opinion disagrees with my doctor's opinion, what should I do?**
  Hopefully, you will know what the second-opinion physician's

recommendation is before you leave her office. If it differs from what your first doctor recommended, say so. Ask the doctor why she is making her recommendation and to compare it to the first physician's recommendation.

This is one of those times when having developed a true partnership with your physician really helps. Remember, the plan is to take the second opinion back to your treating physician. You will discuss the pros and cons just like any other alternative. You are not asking your treating physician to decide between her approach and that of the second physician if they disagree. You are asking the specialist to give you her opinion of what the treating physician recommended. You will have to decide which approach is best for you. In the end, **it may mean that you end up getting treated by the second-opinion doctor or end up going to another physician at a specialized center where certain options are available that your doctor cannot offer you.** If that is best for you, I would expect your doctor to recommend it.

> Take the second opinion back to your treating physician and discuss the pros and cons of it like any other alternative. One option that may have to be considered is transferring your care.

- **Can I use the second-opinion doctor as an ongoing resource?**
  Sometimes the second-opinion specialist will have ideas or perspectives that are beneficial to your overall care. They are not radically different, but you feel they are helpful in getting you the best care. Alternatively, sometimes the second-opinion physician just confirms what your doctor says, but as the disease and treatment process progresses, you begin to desire a follow-up visit to see if the second-opinion doctor is still in agreement. Is that a good idea?

In my experience helping patients navigate through the health-care system, I have found that for some people, there is a definite benefit when the second-opinion doctor plays an intermittent review role.

FOR INSTANCE...

I have a friend, Roger, who has a serious lung disease. He is cared for by an excellent specialist in our hometown. Because of the complexity of Roger's problem, he was referred to a specialist at a local university hospital for a second opinion. This specialist supported the care plan of the first doctor. The second-opinion doctor, in fact, has been very forceful in encouraging my friend to be diligent about following his doctor's instructions.

Roger's condition and treatment has intermittently limited his ability to work. If he works too hard and too long, he often has a flare-up of his condition. When this happens, his doctor adjusts his medicine and gets him to adjust his lifestyle. On more than one occasion during these episodes, Roger has gone back to the university doctor for a follow-up visit. Even though the university doctor has consistently supported the first doctor, the follow-up visits to the second-opinion doctor are very reassuring to him.

10

> Sometimes a follow-up appointment with the second-opinion doctor is helpful as a disease progresses.

• Should I get a third or fourth opinion?

The idea of third or even fourth opinions usually comes to mind if the second opinion does not agree with the first opinion. In most instances, however, getting more opinions is not helpful. **It is tempting to shop until you hear an opinion you like, but it is not wise.** You should follow the course of treatment that is best for you.

In the rare instances where you can not sort out conflicting opinions, you may need the help of a third party. One very good option is to find a physician whom you know and trust and ask him to help you sort out the recommendations. If you have been working with specialists, your primary-care physician can serve in this role. If the issue involves your primary physician and you have no other resource (such as a doctor in the family), then you should consider a third opinion.

I suggest that you seek one of the leading experts in the field at the closest university hospitals. Take your whole dilemma to her. Be totally candid about your conflicting opinions, and see what she says. I would encourage you to make it clear that you are not shopping for opinions; rather you have conflicting recommendations that you can not reconcile without help.

Key Take Home Messages

- A second opinion can be very helpful but it is not necessary in every instance, and it is not always the best for every patient.

- A second opinion can be good reassurance that all alternatives are being explored.

- Take the results of the second opinion back to your treating physician.

- There are times when you will find it best to change your care to the second-opinion doctor.

- There is sometimes a benefit in having intermittent follow-up visits with the second-opinion doctor.

- Avoid shopping for opinions until you hear an opinion you "like." You are looking for the best advice to follow.

11

I'M GOING TO THE HOSPITAL

Where and when should Informed
Consent occur?

What happens if it's an emergency procedure?

What is the usual course of recovery?

What is the likelihood of a
successful outcome?

When should I create advance directives?

Will having advance directives avoid problems?

How can I make sure my desires are
carried through?

Informed Consent: It's Crucial

As your own medical advocate, you want to go to the hospital or prepare for surgery with your eyes wide open—meaning you know exactly what you are getting into. It starts with a **process called Informed Consent.** The critical word here is process. Most people think of Informed Consent as the form you sign to authorize a procedure. It's not. Informed Consent is the discussion your surgeon has with you that leads up to signing the form. By definition, Informed Consent means that you fully understand what to expect before, during, and after surgery. You should not consent to any procedure until this process is accomplished. There are three aspects to Informed Consent:

- Your capacity and freedom to make the choice that is best for you.
- Your understanding of the options being considered.
- Making your decision and formally authorizing the procedure by signing appropriate consent forms.

If your physical or mental capacity is compromised, either by illness or by medications such as painkillers, you may not be fully capable of giving Informed Consent. If you are feeling pressured by family, friends, or your physician to decide in a certain way, this may limit your ability to freely make the choice you want. Recognize that you have the right to decide what you want for yourself. Therefore, you should have this discussion with your doctor when you are physically and emotionally up to making a clear-headed decision.

The discussion itself must accomplish three goals:

- **Disclosure**—Your doctor should disclose to you all the important benefits and risks of the procedure that **he thinks are important for you to know,** and that he thinks you might feel are important, even if he doesn't think they are significant.
- **Recommendation**—Your doctor gives you his recommendation. You are in a partnership with your doctor, and you want his best advice. You cannot be an informed medical advocate and make an informed decision without

knowing what your doctor thinks is best for you.

- **Understanding**—At the end of the discussion, you should understand all the information the doctor has related to you.

There is a difference between disclosure and understanding. It is not enough for your doctor to tell you something, or even to give it to you in writing, if you are left with doubts, questions, or concerns. I believe Informed Consent should be a discussion between the doctor and the patient so the patient has the opportunity to ask questions and get satisfactory answers.

Once you understand what is expected to happen, you can decide if you want to consent to the procedure. If your decision is to go forward, your doctor and the hospital will have forms for you to sign confirming your consent.

> Informed Consent is a discussion your surgeon has with you so you fully understand what to expect.

11

- **Where and when should Informed Consent occur?**
I believe the process of Informed Consent is best **conducted in your doctor's office before you are admitted to the hospital.** This provides time for a thoughtful conversation without the distractions of the hospital environment. It also allows you the option to go home and consider the information before you consent. As soon as your doctor begins discussing a procedure with you, make sure he knows that you want to do the Informed Consent in his office prior to the admission. If he says it is not necessary, tell him you want to do it anyway. You are the person giving the consent…you want the process to work best for you!

- **What happens if it's an emergency procedure?**
Even in emergency situations, the Informed Consent process must take place. You will not have time for a quiet conversation in your doctor's office, but there is usually time to discuss the benefits and risks of the emergency procedure being proposed. If you are incapacitated by illness or injury, your doctor will

obtain consent with the family member closest to you, for instance, your spouse. Only in the most extreme emergencies where delaying the procedure is considered life-or limb-threatening will doctors proceed without Informed Consent.

Asking the Right Questions

Informed Consent can be a stressful conversation, so have your questions prepared in advance. Use the techniques recommended in chapter 4.

- **What is the usual course of recovery?**
  You want to thoroughly understand the procedure you are having, but you also want to know what your recovery will be like. **Everyone recovers from surgery differently, so it is important that you phrase your questions in the right context.**

  > FOR EXAMPLE...
  > If a patient asks a question like, *How soon can I go back to work?* the doctor can honestly say, *I have seen patients back at work in 3 weeks*. This may be true but not the norm. Sure, the doctor has seen patients go back to work in 3 weeks, but the average person is able to return to work in 6 weeks. For others, 12 weeks is more likely. And, it may take a full 6 months before he feels that all his energy has returned.

The doctor does not intend to mislead you. It's just that doctors are more likely to recall their best-case rather than the average-case scenario. Know the difference and ask your doctor the question in three specific ways:

- What is the usual course of recovery?
- What is the best possible course?
- What is the worst possible course?

The usual course is what happens to most patients. Since there is no guarantee you will follow the usual course, you want to know all three. I am not saying that this will always be a comfortable conversation for either you or your doctor, but it is a critical one! I believe recovery is much easier if you know what you are getting into. It is also much easier on family and friends if they are prepared for all possibilities. It also eliminates unnecessary stress if you are not healing as fast as you hoped.

Get the details of the landmarks along the way to your recovery. Ask:

- How long will I be in the hospital?
- How long will I be in bed after I'm home?
- How long will I have pain?
- How long will I be on medication after the surgery?
- When can I resume exercising?
- When can I return to work or my other regular activities?

You can see there are many questions you really want to discuss with your doctor.

> You want to know the usual course as well as the best possible and worst possible course you might experience.

- **What is the likelihood of a successful outcome?**
One technique that often aids in the Informed Consent process is knowing how to **help your doctor give you recovery estimates.**

First, acknowledge that you realize he can not promise you a specific outcome, and say that you just want him to give you his best estimate. If he feels like you are looking for a guaranteed outcome, he will be hesitant to give you any number. This is one of those times you want to be clear with your doctor that you are partners in your care. Tell him that you want the estimates to help prepare yourself, your family, and your friends. If your doctor is confident that you are not trying to back him into a corner, it will be much easier for him to answer your questions more directly.

> Remember, your doctor is giving you an estimate of what the average patient experiences.

Advance Directives

While we all want to believe that we will come through surgery or a hospitalization just fine, the truth is that sometimes things do not always go as hoped. I know from spending years on a hospital medical ethics committee that one of the most important things you can do for yourself and your family is to create and discuss what is called an **advance directive**.

The purpose of an advance directive is to make sure that your wishes regarding your health care are followed in the event that you are unable to express those wishes at some point during your care. Make sure they are clearly communicated in writing, and discuss the contents of the documents fully with your family.

Advance directives usually include three distinct documents: **health care power of attorney, a living will or health care instructions, and a do not resuscitate (DNR) order.** Essentially, these are legal documents that stipulate your desires to your doctors and family. **If you are awake and can communicate, they have no bearing on your care.** However, if you are not, they give guidance as to the care you want and identify whom you wish to speak on your behalf while you are incapacitated.

These documents, and the laws that govern them, can vary from state to state. You can check with your attorney, your doctor, or your hospital for specific information regarding your state. Here is an overview.

Health Care Power of Attorney

This document designates whom you want to make medical decisions and sign medical consents for you if you are incapacitated to do so yourself. This person is called your **health care agent.** You are presumed to be naming someone who will have your best interest at heart, with whom you have discussed these issues, and, most important, who knows what you want and will express these wishes on your behalf. **This**

person should know you well enough to speak to what you would want in any given situation, not what they want for you!

If you do not create a health care power of attorney, the law allows someone to make these decisions on your behalf. The person is usually your spouse or, if you do not have a spouse, your adult children, other family member or close friend. This can create several problems, including:

- The person or persons selected in the absence of an appointed health care agent may not be the person you want making these choices.
- If you have multiple adult children, they all must agree on the decision.
- You are at increased risk of receiving care that you would not have chosen if you were capable of speaking for yourself.

Living Will or Health Care Instructions

11

Stated simply, a **living will** describes specific kinds of medical care you want or do not want. It is only invoked when you are not capable of expressing your own desires. In the state of Maryland where I live, there are three categories of medical conditions that bring the living will into play: A **terminal condition,** where death is believed to be imminent; a **persistent vegetative state,** which has a long, legal definition; and **end stage condition,** in which a person is totally dependent on life-support systems to prevent death.

If you unfortunately end up in any of these conditions, a living will instructs your health-care providers on the measures you do or do not want taken to support your life. Be aware that a living will may be limited to these conditions. Therefore, if a different scenario causes you to end up on a respirator, your living will may not drive the decisions being made. That is why you also want a health care power of attorney.

Do Not Resuscitate Order (DNR)

This is an optional order written by your doctor, with your agreement, that says if you stop breathing or your heart stops, cardio-pulmonary resuscitation (CPR) will not be preformed. It is used for dying patients in the hospital or receiving home care or nursing care. In these latter settings, it spares doctors, nurses, or emergency staff, who are unfamiliar with your wishes, from responding to an emergency.

> AN EXAMPLE OF THIS IS...
> An elderly family member, who was in an advanced stage of dementia, was being cared for in her home by wonderful caregivers. The family and her doctor were aware that, in the case of a medical crisis, heroic measures, including CPR, were not to be used. The caregivers were aware of this, but in order to be sure that there was no confusion, our family had: a posted notice to the caretakers explaining that in the event of a medical crisis, they were to call the doctor, not 911; a medical order written on the doctor's medical stationary for emergency medical technicians in case the caregivers called 911 anyway; and a do not resuscitate order.

My family and the doctor developed a care plan, discussed it with the caregiver, and attempted to document it in written notes and orders for the caregiver or for any other medical providers who might be on the scene.

- **When should I create advance directives?**
  Many people tend to let this go until they or their loved one are facing an end-of-life situation. I can tell you from my years as a clinician as well as from my experience on the medical ethics committee that **the best time to create these documents is when you are well.** It is important to have these documents in place when you are entering a hospital or having surgery or other medical procedures. If something goes wrong and you are incapacitated, it will be left up to your family to decide how your care should be managed. More often than not, this leads to family turmoil and conflict—to put it mildly. I have seen this on numerous occasions, and it is totally avoidable.

- **Will having advance directives avoid problems?**
  There are two common mistakes people make that can create a problem around advanced directives:

  - Not discussing your written desires with all the members of your immediate family.

- Not planning your documents so your family can deal with an unpredicted medical situation.

You need to discuss your wishes with your immediate family. This discussion needs to be complete enough that you and they are comfortable that your desires will be supported when the time comes. Otherwise, **you end up with the scenario where some members of the family want to support your wishes and some do not.**

In this situation, the medical staff may find it very hard to do anything except provide the most conservative care. For instance, let's say the living will that you signed states that you do not want to be on a ventilator if you are comatose. Only, you never discussed it with your family, and then it happens. Some of your family members might push for the ventilator, and some of them might want it turned off. Even if you have a living will, doctors are often loath to turn off the ventilator against the expressed wishes of some family members. If you had discussed your desires with your family, they could uniformly support them.

The second problem families encounter is when a medical situation develops that is not clearly addressed in the advanced directives. You can write your advanced directives to manage the unpredicted, but you will only succeed if you have also discussed this possibility with your family. The conversation regarding your wishes has to be broad enough to cover more than just the predictable possibilities, like being in a coma or on a respirator. The family needs to be able to honestly say that their conversations with you were in depth enough that they understand how you would decide on any medical issues.

For instance, let's say you had multiple rib fractures from which you were expected to make a full recovery, but it requires that you be placed on a ventilator for 2 weeks. Let's say your living will says you do not want to be placed on a ventilator, but your family knows this situation is an exception because your time on the ventilator will be limited and a full recovery is anticipated. When you write your living will, you should state your preferences as guiding principles. However, you should also state that your health care agent has the authority to make

11

the final decision for you, even if it conflicts with your living will. You should also place similar wording in the health care power of attorney so the health care agent is empowered to make medical decisions on your behalf after he considers the situation.

> Advance directives can save your family a great amount of emotional turmoil and give you peace of mind that your wishes will be followed.

- **How can I make sure my desires are carried through?**
  Your most powerful tool is to make sure that there is official written documentation of your desires and that they have been conveyed to your family through conversation.

  Advance directives are always difficult issues to think about, and many of us say we are going to do them, but fail to do so. Don't wait any longer.

Key Take Home Messages

- True Informed Consent is a conversation between you and your doctor.

- Know the difference among the usual course of recovery, the best course, and a complicated course.

- Get the details on recovery landmarks.

- Discuss your wishes for medical care with your family and document them in advance directives.

12

I'M IN THE HOSPITAL!

How can my medical advocate help keep
a medication mistake from happening to me?

What can my medical advocate do to
protect me from getting a hospital-borne infection?

What should we do if my medical advocate
feels intimidated by the hospital staff?

Am I being a burden?

What if my spouse is also ill or not strong
enough to help me?

Never Be Alone

I believe without question that for major illnesses or surgeries, the best place to be is in the hospital. I also believe that you never want to spend a moment alone in the hospital as a patient. Never, never, never! Someone should be with you at all times to serve as your medical advocate.

Don't get me wrong. This is not an indictment of hospitals, doctors, and nurses. I believe that people who take up the medical profession do so because they want to help others. Hospital staffs are dedicated and caring. They work hard. But hospitals everywhere are short-staffed because there is a shortage of registered nurses—not only in America but worldwide—and it is expected to continue for years.

The care in a hospital is complex, and the staffs are often overworked. **Mistakes do happen, even under the best of conditions, and they happen more often than you might believe.** This is why you need to be an informed and observant patient. It's also why you need someone with you at all times. You don't want a mistake to happen to you. In many instances, they are easy to avoid.

> You never, never, never want to spend a moment alone in the hospital!

CONSIDER, FOR INSTANCE, THIS EXAMPLE...
When my daughter was a teenager, she was admitted to the hospital during the middle of the night with a diagnosis of appendicitis. The surgeon diagnosed her in the emergency room and suggested waiting a few hours to see how her symptoms progressed to be sure the diagnosis was correct. Meanwhile, he told us that he scheduled surgery for 7:30 A.M., but would re-examine her to confirm the diagnosis. My daughter was transferred to a hospital room, and I settled into a reclining chair next to her bed for the night.

Around 7:00 A.M., two orderlies from the operating room came to get her for surgery. I explained that the surgeon said he was planning to see her to confirm her diagnosis before the final decision to operate would be made. They said they had been told to take her to the O.R. and proceeded to try to do so. I politely but clearly said they needed to contact the surgeon and remind him that he had planned to re-examine her first. A few minutes later, the surgeon arrived, dressed in his scrubs. He repeated his exam and was surprised (and frustrated) to discover that my daughter's medical condition had not progressed as he had expected. In fact, the location and nature of her pain and tenderness had changed.

Visibly upset with this development, the surgeon explained that it no longer appeared that my daughter had appendicitis. It turns out that she had a nonsurgical problem that would resolve on its own.

The lesson in this story is clear. **The advocate is there to be sure that important steps don't get missed.**

12

How Errors Happen

The role of your medical advocate is to help prevent hospital errors from happening to you; it's a role that can literally save your life. This is not an overstatement. Let's look at the risk of avoidable injury while in the hospital, according to the most recent statistics.

- Three out of 100 patients in a hospital experience an avoidable medical error.
- One out of 200 will die as a result of an avoidable error.

There are several types of avoidable hospital errors including:

- Incorrect medications and dosages
- Missed medications
- Surgical errors
- Hospital-acquired infections
- Errors in nursing care

> There are a large number of
> avoidable injuries and deaths
> each year from hospital errors.

Mix-Ups in Medications

The most common type of errors in the hospital involves medications. **One study found that patient drugs were administered
incorrectly 19 percent of the time,** with 7 percent of the errors
having potentially harmful consequences. Of the 19 percent:

- 43 percent of patients were given their medicine at the
  wrong time
- 30 percent were not given their medicine
- 17 percent received the wrong dose
- 4 percent were given the wrong medication

> Medication errors happen,
> but they are preventable.

Another study found that 54 percent of patients failed to
continue to get their routine medicine at least once during their
hospitalization. Of these errors, 38 percent had the potential to
cause moderate to severe harm.

> HERE IS AN EXAMPLE OF HOW AN ACCIDENT CAN
> HAPPEN—AND BE AVOIDED...
> A nurse came into a woman's hospital room and handed
> her a pill and a cup of water. The patient said she did not
> recognize the medicine and wanted to know what it was.
> The nurse said it was a diuretic, and her doctor wanted her
> to take it. The woman insisted that her doctor had not told
> her anything about taking the pill and refused to take it.
> Finally, the nurse said, "Now, Mrs. Smith, there is no
> mistake. Your doctor wants you to take this." As you can
> probably guess, the patient was not Mrs. Smith. Her
> persistence paid off.

The lesson here is that you must hold your ground. Ask the nurse what pill she is giving you, and if you are unaware that you should be taking it, don't take it. Get confirmation from your doctor first.

- **How can my medical advocate help keep a medication mistake from happening to me?**
This is a particularly important role for your medical advocate. Often, the patient in the hospital is not fully oriented. The medical advocate can be the observer when the patient can not.

When you go to the hospital, **have a written list of what medications you are on** and what you should be continuing to take while you are in the hospital. Share it with your medical advocate. Here are some of the key things you or your advocate can do:

- Make sure the floor nurses have a list of your routine medications that you are to continue while in the hospital.
- Obtain the list of medications your doctor has ordered for you while in the hospital.
- Talk to your doctor if any routine medications are missing from the hospital list.
- Check the medication, timing, and dosage of each medication the nurse brings you. If there is an error, speak up.
- Call the nurse if a scheduled medicine is late.

12

> You and your medical advocate need to know and monitor the medications you are given in the hospital.

Surgery—Which Side?

There have been well-publicized stories of errors in which a surgeon operates on the wrong knee (or other body part) or even performs a surgery on the wrong patient. These types of errors are rare, but you don't want one to happen to you. The cautious medical advocate can take steps to avoid these types of errors.

> **FOR INSTANCE . . .**
> My neighbor Judy was having hip surgery and wanted to make sure the surgeon operated on the correct hip. She was told to write "OPERATE HERE" on the correct side, but she didn't think this was enough. She also wrote "WRONG SIDE" on her other hip. She knew that she would be covered with surgical drapes in the operating room and one hip would never be seen by the surgical team. With instructions on both hips, she figured there would be no mistake!

The lesson here is that there is no such thing as being too careful when you are in the hospital. Your medical advocate can't be with you in the operating room, but she can help you to remember to cover all your bases.

> Once in the operating room, make sure someone checks your I.D. bracelet to confirm that you are the patient they expected.

Hospital-Acquired Infections

One of the risks of being in the hospital is the possibility of getting a hospital-borne infection. Hospital infections are called **nosocomial infections** and are more common than most people appreciate. This is a significant problem for doctors and hospitals. In fact, hospitals have special committees and protocols to track and try to prevent these infections because, unfortunately, they can be quite serious.

Nosocomial infections can occur for many reasons, surgical and nonsurgical. Sometimes there is a break in sterile procedures in the operating room; sometimes there is a break in technique in changing surgical dressing. Often, though, we never know the cause.

What we do know is that infections acquired in the hospital

are often harder to treat than infections acquired outside the hospital. This is due to more than just the patient's weakened state. It is the unfortunate truth that the organisms that cause hospital-acquired infections are frequently more dangerous than those encountered outside the hospital. The high usage of antibiotics in the hospital results in more resistant strains of bacteria. This means that the treatment is often more difficult, and the chance of the infection killing the patient is greater.

- **What can my medical advocate do to protect me from getting a hospital-borne infection?**
  Although there is no guarantee that the medical advocate can prevent nosocomial infections, there are things she can do to decrease the risks. A few of them are:

  - Make sure that anyone, including doctors and nursing staff, who touches the patient washes their hands first.
  - Make sure that surgical dressings are changed on schedule.
  - Make sure there is not an accidental exposure to infection by means of a minor procedure such as an IV or a urinary catheter. For instance, a nurse handling a catheter may not notice it brushing against a nonsterile bed sheet. If you or your advocate notices anything like this, speak up.
  - Your advocate can encourage you to be as active as your doctor allows. She can assist your efforts to be out of bed and walking as much as allowed.
  - If your doctor has ordered you to have respiratory therapy or use devices to encourage deep breathing, your advocate can make sure you use them as directed.

> Hospital-acquired infections are a major threat to patients. Your medical advocate needs to have this in mind.

12

The Importance of Having an Advocate

To suggest that someone be in the hospital with a patient at all times strikes many people as impossible and perhaps a bit ludicrous. It is not. Obviously, doing so requires the help of more than one person. I suggest a small team of family and close friends who can rotate being with you. **Someone should even spend the night with you.** At night, hospital staffing is at its lowest, and, therefore, the risk of something going wrong is the highest.

Your advocate's primary duty is to understand the care you should receive and also what you should not receive. I see your advocate approaching this in two roles: offensive and defensive.

The **offensive role** is to be your arms and legs and voice when you are limited by your illness or surgery. You need someone to hand you things, to go looking for the nurse if you ring the call button and no one answers, to make sure you get your meals, to walk the halls with you if you are able, and so on. Your advocate can make telephone calls on your behalf to let people know how you are doing. Basically, this person is an extension of you when you are limited.

The **defensive role** is to be sure that nothing happens to you in the hospital that your doctor has not ordered. This includes making sure you are getting the proper medications, tests, and treatments your doctor has scheduled for you. Your advocate should keep track of any consultants your doctor said would be seeing you that day. Also, if you are scheduled for x-rays, physical therapy, respiratory therapy, or any of the other many services your doctor may have ordered, your advocate should make sure those happen on schedule as well.

Your advocate's defensive role **should not create an adversarial relationship with the hospital staff.** Rather, it is recognition that mistakes can happen, but that vigilance can avoid them. Your advocate does need to be alert and assertive on your behalf without being aggressive. It is important that there be no confusion or disagreement between your understanding of what should happen and what is happening.

- **What should we do if my medical advocate feels intimidated by the hospital staff?**

Neither you nor your advocate should ever allow yourselves to be intimidated by the hospital staff. You want to persist in questioning what and why they are proposing something until it is consistent with the care plan as you understand it. Your advocate can and must do this for you, if you are not feeling well enough to handle it yourself.

> The role of a medical advocate is not an adversarial one.

A GOOD EXAMPLE...

To say that my close friend, George, had major surgery is putting it mildly. He was heavily bandaged and medicated when we went to see him the evening of his surgery. At about 8:30 P.M., George's wife went into the bathroom in his hospital room and changed into her pajamas. She announced that she planned to spend the night with him, and intended to stay for as long as the hospitalization lasted. As we were saying our good-byes, she climbed into bed next to George. A nurse arrived at about that time, and, as you can imagine, the nurse was adamant that his wife could not sleep in the bed with him. My friend's wife was equally adamant that she was not moving. She said she would be extremely careful not to disturb the surgical area, but that she planned to be close to him to provide him with the love and comfort he received at home. She won!

12

Now I am not proposing sleeping in the patient's bed as everyone's strategy. However, it does show how loved ones can provide emotional and physical support, even in an acute-care hospital.

Everyone wants to be helpful when you or a loved one is ill, and very few know what to do. I believe asking someone to be part of your medical advocate team is a real gift to them. They can contribute to your recovery! What nicer role could they hope to play? Here are a few other things your advocate can do:

- **Monitor your visitors.** Visitors can be the best or the worst part of your hospital experience. You may want family and friends around, and you should encourage them to visit, but it is your advocate's job to try and coordinate your visitations. If you are not up for visitors, your advocate can be the one to encourage a short visit or politely let someone know it is time to leave.

- **Make sure you get your rest.** A hospital is not the place for you to have to entertain visitors. You need your rest and strength to heal. You need to watch how you are holding up with visitations and candidly guide your medical advocate on your needs.

- **Play host.** Hospital visits can be filled with a lot of awkward moments. Your advocate can host the visitors and carry the conversation, so you don't have to. Your advocate can also let your visitors know that it is okay to sit beside you and hold your hand. Personal contact is an amazing recovery tool that people tend to shy away from when they are visiting someone who is ill.

- **Bring you meals.** Nourishment is an important part of healing but hospitals are notorious for serving less-than-tasty food. If your doctor has not placed you on a restricted diet, there is no reason you have to eat the hospital's food. Again, ask your doctor—not the floor nurse. A nice thing to ask friends to do is to bring you meals. This is a good chore for your advocate to coordinate. It is amazing how good food can make a hospital stay much more bearable.

> Too much of a good thing can be bad for anyone, and that includes too many visitors.

A Shared Experience

We all have people who want to provide help and support when we're in need, be it family, friends, or both. This is your medical advocate team, and it is a good thing to have. It is not a weakness to depend on others when you are incapacitated. I believe it is weakness to be afraid to ask for help. Even if you go through an illness seemingly asking little from those around you, your illness has an impact on your family and friends. Accept their gift of caring by letting them help you. You are the patient, but they are sharing your medical experience in their own way.

• Am I being a burden?

How often have you said or heard this? Recognize that letting your loved ones help you and share some of your burden is a gift. We seem to know this when someone else is the patient, but fail to acknowledge it when we are the one in need. Most people feel helpless when a loved one is sick and have a hard time figuring out how they can help. The best gift you can give your loved ones is to tell them your needs. I sometimes think patients become a burden because they stubbornly insist that they do not need help.

• What if my spouse is also ill or not strong enough to help me?

The capacity of your support system is an important thing for you to consider early in any illness.

12

> FOR EXAMPLE...
> I knew an elderly couple who both needed to use walkers to get around. When the husband got ill and grew weaker, his wife, with her walker, would walk behind his walker in case he lost his balance. What a loving and sweet act! But if he fell, she could fall, too.

Support systems sometimes need their own support. Do a frank appraisal of the support you will need and where you believe it will come from. Planning in advance can avoid a very stressful period for everyone.

You and others on your team should recognize that **your primary caregiver will need time to refill her tank.** This is an opportunity for others to step in who want to help.

> Often the best gift the patient can give her loved ones is to tell them what she needs.

Bother Your Doctor—It's Her Job!

Your doctor is the head of your health-care team and, as your medical partner, should be aware of all the care you are getting while you are in the hospital. She should be discussing your care and progress with you and your advocate. If something in your care seems inappropriate or not what you understood should take place, do not allow it. Ask to speak to your doctor.

Many patients have told me that they "hate to bother the doctor." I believe **there is no such thing as bothering your doctor.** If you think a medication is wrong and the nurse disagrees with you, tell her you want to talk to your doctor before you proceed. If the nurse returns and says she has spoken with your doctor, tell her you want to speak with your doctor. If something doesn't seem right, you should not surrender until you hear it is okay directly from your doctor.

> A GOOD EXAMPLE...
> When my daughter Amy was having throat surgery, her doctor told her that her mother and I would be there when she woke up in the recovery room. Around the expected time, we got a call from the doctor that surgery had just ended, and all was well. I asked if we could go to the recovery room then. He said the staff needed a few minutes to get our daughter settled, and they would call us. No call came. My wife suggested that I call the doctor and find out why they hadn't called. I am sorry to say, I was hesitant to "bother" him. So we waited. Eventually, they called, but long after our daughter was awake. When she woke up and did not find us by her side, she was upset and thought it meant that something had gone wrong.

This shows how hard it sometimes is to "bother" the doctor. I had guessed he was back in the O.R. doing his next surgery. It shouldn't have mattered to me. Don't let it matter to you. The medical advocate has to stay focused on the task at hand, which is to speak to the best interests of the patient. The system will take care of itself!

It's okay to bother your doctor. She is your health-care partner. You need to feel comfortable talking with her when you need to.

Key Take Home Messages

- You never, never, never want to be alone in the hospital!

- You need a medical advocate who can support your needs in a nonadversarial way.

- You and your medical advocate need to know and monitor your medications.

- Don't consent to something without knowing for sure it was authorized by your doctor.

- If you don't have to eat the hospital food, have your meals brought in.

- There is no such thing as bothering your doctor.

12

13

WHEN THE DOCTOR SAYS "SURGERY"

Why is it major surgery if it is happening to me?

How does more information help me?

Does surgery always help?

When is the best time to schedule surgery?

How do I know if I have a good surgeon?

Do I have a choice between outpatient and inpatient surgery?

There's No Such Thing as Minor Surgery

I have a strong viewpoint when it comes to having surgery that I recommend every medical advocate adopt: **It may be minor surgery to the doctor, but it is major surgery if it is happening to me**! I assure you that your doctor is not using this definition. Whether he calls it major or minor, you should always view it as major. It's the best way to protect your health.

> It is major surgery if it is being done to me; it is minor surgery if it is being done to someone else!

LET ME SHARE THE EXAMPLE OF ONE OF MY GRANDSONS...

At 4 months of age, doctors discovered that some of the bones in his skull had fused prematurely. This meant that his brain would not continue its normal growth unless the bones were separated. His pediatrician reassured my daughter that this was relatively minor surgery. Fortunately, we live close to a university that has one of the world's best pediatric neurosurgeons, so we scheduled an appointment for a second opinion. He saw my grandson, and he agreed that surgery was necessary. My daughter remembers the neurosurgeon telling her that, compared to the surgeries he usually does, this was relatively minor. I will spare you the details except to say that my grandson was on a ventilator for over 12 hours, in the pediatric intensive care unit for 2 days, and in the hospital for 5 days. I know that this really was a relatively minor procedure to the surgeon; however, to the baby, the parents, and the grandparents, I assure you this was major surgery.

A Difference in Perspective

To be fair, I believe that your doctor almost always is trying to communicate the truth to you. By almost, I mean he also does not want to frighten you unnecessarily. However, as discussed in chapter 11, I think that **doctors unconsciously tend to discuss their surgeries based on their best outcomes as opposed to their most common ones.**

• **Why is it major surgery if it is happening to me?**
First of all, essentially there is nothing done in medicine that doesn't carry some risk. There is no surgery that doesn't have a potential downside. Does that mean you shouldn't have surgery? Not at all. However, I believe that agreeing to something that carries an inherent risk is a major decision. Therefore, any surgery I agree to undergo is major surgery.

It means that you want to have meaningful conversations with your doctor so you understand what the usual—that is, the most common—outcome is and what the possible exceptions are. This is the "Informed Consent" that I discussed in chapter 11. It is worth rereading any time your doctor suggests surgery.

• **How does more information help me?**
By understanding the true nature of a surgery, including all its risks and benefits, you can better decide if it is in your best interest to have it done.

13

TAKE, FOR EXAMPLE...
An older man whose prostate is enlarged and who is getting up two or three times a night to go to the bathroom goes to his doctor and complains about his interrupted sleep. The doctor refers him to an urologist. The urologist examines him and says that his prostate is enlarged and that this problem can be corrected by a TURP (transurethral resection of the prostate). The man schedules the surgery.

Now, if the man is also told that 3 to 5 percent of patients who have TURPs end up with urinary incontinence (a loss of some of the voluntary control of the bladder), and if he is told, in addition, that at this point in his care, the enlarged prostate is not a threat to his overall health—except for the nightly interruptions—would he still schedule the surgery?

Maybe so, but maybe not. He did go to the doctor complaining about having to get up at night, so he may feel the risk is worth it. He may decide that, to him, a 3 to 5 percent risk of incontinence is worse than having to go to the bathroom 2 or 3 times a night. Or he may decide that the inconvenience of getting up at night is better than having to go through surgery. He may decide he can put off the decision until he starts having to get up seven or eight times a night. He might also ask his doctor about alternative strategies and learn that if he limits what he drinks after 7:00 P.M., he could cut down on his trips to the bathroom.

I do not think his doctor is lying to him or intentionally withholding information. The doctor heard the man's complaint and offered a solution. The enlightened medical advocate, however, will realize that the physician's first recommendation to solving a problem might not be the patient's first choice.

The issue at hand is what may be the right decision for one person may be the wrong decision for another. Only the patient can decide what he considers a major inconvenience. Only the patient can decide what feels like a major risk and if that risk is worth taking.

You need to get all the necessary information and understand all the options to make the best decision. You must consider it from your own perspective, not your doctor's or someone else's.

> What may be the right decision for one person might be the wrong decision for another.

• Does surgery always help?

Nothing always helps. However, your surgeon can guide you with numbers on the probability of it helping. He can also guide you on what the likelihood of different outcomes are. For instance, he should be able to tell you the percentage of complete cure versus the percentage of improvement without a complete cure. Different doctors have different perspectives on surgery.

FOR INSTANCE...

I know a neurosurgeon who has a terrific success rate on performing disc surgery and getting significant pain relief for his patients. I asked him why his patients always seem

> to get pain relief, while other surgeons don't seem to have
> such a high success rate. His answer was simple, "I don't
> operate unless I am sure it will take away the pain."

Now, this is not a condemnation of other surgeons. But it is an example of how different surgeons have their own way of doing their jobs. You could say that with an attitude like the surgeon in the example, some patients who might benefit from surgery would not get it because he wasn't "sure" it would help. What it teaches us is that we want to know how our surgeon views the potential and probable outcomes. Only then can we decide whether or not to have surgery, when, and by whom.

Timing Can Be Everything

Surgery is divided into three categories and, as your own medical advocate, you should understand the difference among them.

Emergency surgery means that you are in imminent danger of losing life or limb if you don't have surgery now. Examples of this type of surgery include an appendectomy, some heart surgeries for patients who have had heart attacks, and surgeries that are needed as a result of a serious injury or accident. With emergency surgery, the only discussion of timing is "how quickly."

Elective surgery means that there is no threat to life, limb, or longevity. It is surgery that if you choose not to have it, it will not significantly compromise your health. The most common example of elective surgery is cosmetic surgery.

Surgery is called **semi-elective** when it is needed to correct or avoid some functional impairment, but it is not necessary to avoid an immediate threat to your health or life. A good example is hip-replacement surgery for degenerative arthritis. You may want the surgery so you will not be incapacitated or limited in your lifestyle. The big question is *When should you have the surgery?* This is something to which you need to give careful thought and consideration.

Surgery is not something I encourage people to volunteer for unless and until it is necessary. **If it is necessary, then do it when you feel it is warranted, and not before.**

> FOR INSTANCE...
> I know a man who was told his kidneys were beginning to fail. He was told he would likely need either renal (kidney) dialysis or a kidney transplant in about a year. He figured why wait a year if he was eventually going to need it anyway? Why not get it done and over with?
>
> When he posed these questions to me, I suggested that he might want to slow down a bit. Dialysis is challenging because it must be done several times a week. Plus, it has its own list of possible medical complications.
>
> So, I understand why he wanted a kidney transplant instead. However, a kidney transplant also has a list of risks and problems. I told him the ideal time to get the transplant would be the day before his doctor said he needed to start dialysis. He considered my advice and decided to wait.

The irony of this story is that well over a year later he was no closer to needing the surgery than the day we had our discussion. The point is this: Do not volunteer for surgery unless and until you really need it. Talk to your doctor about the benefits or risks of waiting to have the surgery.

- **When is the best time to schedule surgery?**
  When scheduling surgery, there are a few things to keep in mind.

> TAKE THIS STORY AS AN EXAMPLE...
> When my 4-month-old grandson needed skull surgery, it was unfortunately scheduled for June 30. I say unfortunately because at university hospitals like the one in which my grandson had surgery, new interns begin on July 1st. Of course, this should have occurred to me beforehand, but in the emotions of the moment, it did not. It wasn't until after the surgery, when this infant was in the pediatric intensive care unit and on a respirator, that I realized our bad timing.

> We could hear the good-bye party for the interns taking place in the nurses' station. The next morning, brand-new interns fresh out of medical school would become part of my infant grandson's health-care team.

Now I want to be clear that he received superb care throughout his stay in the hospital. However, had we planned better, we might have suggested somewhat different timing. It might not have been possible, but at least it would have been discussed.

The point is that there are times when having surgery are less than optimum, as in the case of my grandson. If possible, avoid being in the hospital over major holidays, when staffing is lowest. Also, make sure that your surgeon isn't going on vacation or going to be out of town after your surgery. You want your surgeon to be there to manage your care, especially if something unexpected occurs.

Also, think about your own schedule and the schedules of the people who will be assisting you in your recovery. Find out how much time you will need to recover. (You will find out more details about this in chapter 14). One thing about elective or semi-elective surgery is that you can often pretty much elect to have it at your convenience.

13

> Timing can be everything—talk to your doctor about the optimal time to have planned surgery.

Blood Transfusions—Is There a Risk?

In this time of AIDS and other communicable diseases, many people are concerned about the possibility of getting tainted blood should they need a transfusion during surgery. This is something I encourage you to discuss with your doctor. Let me say that **I think we have an extremely fine blood-testing and blood-banking system in the United States.** Nevertheless, many people are uncomfortable about receiving a transfusion from an unknown donor. If there is a possibility that you will need a transfusion, there are other options.

The safest blood to get is your own blood. Hospital blood banks are set up to draw blood from you and store it in advance of elective surgery. By the time surgery occurs, your body will have replaced the blood that was drawn by the blood bank, and your blood counts will be back to normal. The blood you deposited in the blood bank will be ready should you need a transfusion during surgery.

The other option is to **ask family and friends who have the same blood type as you to donate blood for you.** There are differences of opinions about whether this is any safer than taking the blood available from the blood bank. This is something I encourage you to discuss with your doctor.

> Talk to your doctor about the possibility and options regarding blood transfusions.

The Watch-and-Wait Approach

In chapter 1, I discussed my own case of the still-unknown lesion in my brain, and the decision my doctors and I made about taking the watch-and-wait approach. There are obvious pluses and minuses to this approach—specifically, your doctor is doing the watching, but you are doing the waiting. This approach is a good option only if both you and your physician believe there is no risk of something happening that will change your eventual outcome.

FOR EXAMPLE...

In my instance, my doctor decided that he would monitor me very closely at first (initially every 2 weeks), and then gradually increase the intervals between testing for any change. If a change was found, it would not have had sufficient time to grow into the range that would put me in jeopardy. While the watch-and-wait approach has the wonderful advantage of potentially avoiding surgery, you do pay an emotional price for it.

Waiting sounds easier than it is. You always seem to have

> this thought in the back of your mind, *Is it growing?* To the
> credit of my neurosurgeon, he had a very straightforward
> conversation with me about the emotional toll of waiting.
> Although he recommended this course of treatment, he
> told me that if the waiting made me too anxious or
> depressed, we should re-evaluate the plan.

This approach is not the best for everyone, even if it is offered.
It is also not appropriate for every medical condition. It only
applies when your doctor believes that you do not need
emergency treatment and that "watching" will not lead to
changes that will compromise your ability to be cured. It also
only applies if the patient is comfortable with the process.

How to Choose a Surgeon

This is one of the areas where you want to be a diligent medical
advocate! In some ways, this decision is similar to how you pick
your primary-care provider as we discussed in chapter 2.
However, there are key differences. In picking a surgeon (or
other specialist), look to your primary-care physician for a
recommendation. You also want to ask why he chose that
surgeon.

> You want a surgeon who is
> experienced in your procedure
> and does it often enough to
> keep his skills optimal.

- **How do I know if I have a good surgeon?**
  There are some key questions you should ask the surgeon
  about his history with the surgery you will be having. **How many
  similar surgeries has the surgeon performed?** Though there is no
  hard-and-fast rule, **I personally like my surgeon to have done at
  least ten of the surgeries before operating on me.**

  How often does he perform this surgery? Again there is no set
  rule, and it varies somewhat by how common the surgery is.

I believe it's best if the surgeon does the operation at least once a month. If you can find one who does it once a week, all the better.

Same-Day Surgery

Ambulatory surgery centers, where patients check in and check out the same day, have revolutionized medicine. Though they create some inconvenience for the patient, they **are set up to be every bit as good as a hospital operating room.** The bonus is that you don't have to check into a hospital room.

The driving force behind the expansion of outpatient surgery has been the pressure to control medical costs. By having the patient go home directly from the surgical recovery room, overall medical expenses are lower. This has been driven largely by insurance companies that are increasingly refusing to pay for inpatient surgery unless there is a medical reason why outpatient surgery is not acceptable. Notice the determination is based on the medical necessity of staying in the hospital, not its supportive role.

Outpatient surgery centers are set up to manage less-complicated surgeries. They consist of pre-operative areas, where the patient is prepared for surgery; the operating rooms, where surgery takes place; and a recovery room where the patient is cared for immediately after surgery. The recovery room is where the patient wakes up and rests until he is ready to leave the surgical center. If you have inpatient surgery, you go from the recovery room to your hospital bed. These centers can be in the hospital, off-site but associated with the hospital, or independently owned by other parties.

The operation and the recovery room experience should be the same for the patient whether it is inpatient or outpatient. The post-operative recovery process will not be, and this is the heart of great debate. For the patient, the difference is recovering in the hospital amidst a professional medical staff, or recovering at home on your own with the help of family, friends, or a visiting nurse.

- **Do I have a choice between outpatient and inpatient surgery?**

  If you are having any kind of surgery (which, remember, is always major to you) that does not require a hospital stay, you will most likely have it done on an outpatient basis. You will only be admitted to the hospital if your medical condition warrants it. For you, the patient, this is both good news and bad.

  It is good news because while being in the hospital is the best place to be if you need a professional level of care, it is not the best place to be if you don't. Plus, the staffs at surgical centers are specially trained to transition you right from the recovery room to your car and driver. You are in safe hands.

  The bad news is that you are sent home in a partially medicated state with no professional nurses and other hospital staff to care for you.

  If you are having outpatient surgery, **there are differences in the preparation you need to make in your support system.** Once you wake up in the recovery room, it isn't long before you are out the door and on your way home. This transition can feel so much more abrupt than if you have been in the hospital after surgery and have experienced your post-operative condition in the supportive environment of the hospital. This means you will need to have your home prepared to receive you in your expected post-operative state before you leave for the ambulatory surgery center. The details of what to expect and what to do are covered in the next chapter.

13

Children and Surgery

Many of the surgeries children undergo are done in an outpatient facility. These include tonsil surgery and putting ear tubes in children who have repeated ear infections. I believe **children, like adults, do better if they are well-prepared for the event.**

Naturally, this will vary with the age of the child. In general, if the child is old enough to understand the event, I suggest you make a visit with your child to the facility in advance of the surgery. In the same way that pregnant mothers often visit the labor-and-delivery suites, I believe that taking your child to the facility will provide him some level of comfort on the day of surgery as he will have been there before.

The parent should talk to the anesthesiologist before surgery to find out about the choices in anesthesia. Ask your pediatrician to help you schedule this conversation. Also ask your pediatrician for a recommendation, and ask why. It is extremely important to discuss the steps the facility will take to decrease your child's anxiety, particularly as the procedure is getting started. Can you be there with your child as they put him to sleep?

> Discuss in advance all the steps the facility takes to decrease your child's anxiety.

A very important moment is when your child wakes up from anesthesia. Some recovery rooms are set up to have the parents at the bedside as the child awakens. If this is not the routine at the facility you are using, ask for an exception to allow you to be there. This can be very important, even for older children. They are used to looking to their parents for safety. You want them to see you as they awaken so you can reassure them that all is well. This conversation needs to be held in advance and reaffirmed just before surgery. If you encounter resistance, push through it!

Key Take Home Messages

- Major surgery is when it is done to me; minor surgery is when it is done to someone else!

- You need to ask all the right questions and get specific answers before deciding if you want surgery, and if you want it now.

- You are the final word on whether or not you will have surgery.

- Surgery does not always help—know the risks and benefits.

- Inpatient and outpatient surgery is the same; it is the recovery that is different.

- Don't ask to be admitted to the hospital if it is not necessary.

- Children, like adults, do better if they are well-prepared for surgery.

- Plan to be with your child when he wakes up in the recovery room.

RECOVERY TAKES TIME

How long will it take to heal?

Will I have a lot of pain?

Why am I so tired?

Why must someone accompany
me to outpatient surgery?

Is it really necessary to have someone
do everything for me?

What other things should I do to prepare
for my recovery?

Know Before You Undergo

Whether you are recovering from surgery or an illness, healing takes time. The quickness of your recovery can not be predetermined as a certain number of weeks or months.I believe that **no matter how fast you recover, it will feel like a slow process.**

Typically, the sicker you are, the longer it takes; however, even a mild illness takes time to get over. **Most surgeries take 3 to 6 months for a full recovery.** My rule-of-thumb is that you can expect to be dragging for up to 2 weeks as a result of the anesthesia, even if you are under for only a short period of time. There are countless limitations that must be dealt with when you are recovering from an illness. You may have to face prolonged occupational therapy or go through extensive physical therapy. The list is endless. The important thing is to recognize that healing and recovery take time. Patience isn't just a virtue, it is a requirement!

> Healing and recovery after surgery or an illness take time.

Ask Your Doctor for Guidelines

Your doctor should be your prime source for information on what you should expect after surgery, and it is something you should discuss with her beforehand. **I believe you should be very assertive in working with your doctor to define realistic expectations.** Again, this is a place where you may have to work with your doctor to get her best estimation of your probable course of recovery. As we already discussed, if she feels you are asking for a guarantee, you will not get one. Remember, the way to ask is:

- What is the best I can expect?
- What is the worst I can expect?
- What is most common?

If you are clear that you understand that she is making an educated guess, then she can guide you from her experience with prior similar patients.

- **How long will it take to heal?**
  This is a critical question that, unfortunately, does not have a simple answer. **There are many aspects to healing, and you need to look at them individually.** These are the important things you want to know:

  - How long will I be in the hospital?
  - How long will I have to convalesce at home?
  - How long before I can drive a car?
  - When can I go back to work?
  - When can I resume exercise?
  - How long will it take to get my energy back?
  - How do I deal with the stitches?
  - How common is post-operative depression after my type of surgery?

  If you are having elective or semi-elective surgery, the answers to these questions are important in deciding when to schedule surgery. Keep in mind, though, that you are dealing with estimated timeframes.

14

- **Will I have a lot of pain?**
  You have to expect some discomfort and even some pain, but usually pain will resolve relatively quickly. This varies with your condition. If you are in pain, tell your doctor. **Significant pain is not necessary.** Pain can be managed with medication without harming you. For most people, it is fatigue, rather than pain, that drags on.

- **Why am I so tired?**
  After surgery, people are often surprised by how long it takes to get their full energy back. Many, if not most, people can feel low on energy for up to 6 months. Though the reasons for fatigue are not fully understood, part is attributed to the body using its resources to heal tissue damaged in surgery. This is not a reason to not have surgery. It simply means that

you should **expect to be dragging for some time and to plan your life for the near future with this in mind.** It also means that you have to allow yourself to be tired and to rest without worrying that something about the surgery has gone wrong. If you are concerned about the degree of tiredness, call your doctor.

> There are many different aspects to healing. You need to look at all of them and how they will impact your life.

You also need to be prepared mentally. Although you may go into the surgery feeling rested and strong, you will most likely come out of surgery feeling tired and weak, and quite possibly still somewhat groggy. If you do not know to expect this, it can be very stressful when it happens.

Preparing Yourself and Your Home for Your Recovery

Preparing your home for your return from the hospital is always important, but it is essential to have all contingencies covered when you are returning home after having surgery. This is particularly important if you are having outpatient surgery.

- **Why must someone accompany me to outpatient surgery?**
  Although you might be able to drive yourself to the surgery, you will not be allowed to drive yourself home. **Have someone go with you, stay there with you, drive you home, and stay with you for at least a day afterward.**

  You will probably be very sleepy from the sedation or anesthesia used during the surgery. It is unlikely that you will be in any shape to cook your own meals, much less manage any medicines you need to take. Make sure that all post-operative instructions are written down (they usually are) so your caregiver knows what you need.

It is important that someone be there who can call the doctor in the event that you experience a complication or other unexpected problem. Your caregiver can observe and relate any changes in your behavior or wound that you may not notice.

When your caregiver needs to leave for a short time or to go to work, plan to have your family and friends visit during these times. They can also bring you things you need, including a few groceries or your prescription refills.

> Have someone with you the day of your surgery and plan for a support team during your recovery at home.

• Is it really necessary to have someone do everything for me?

For any kind of significant illness or surgery, you will be out of commission for some period of time. You will make your recovery much easier if you **plan in advance for who will perform your routine chores** while you are recovering. Planning means more than just having someone lined up to take care of you. It means going over the tasks someone will need to do for you, from taking out the trash to doing the laundry to paying your bills on time. Make lists of things that need to be done in advance and go over them with your designated caregiver.

14

This applies to home and work. While you are recovering, you will not be in the mood, nor will you have the energy and focus, to answer questions or remember things that should not be overlooked. If you are prepared in advance, you will save yourself a major hassle!

> Prepare your home and work for your absence.

• What other things should I do to prepare for my recovery?

There may be some physical limitations after your surgery. Consider the following:

- **If you have a two-story home, will you be able to walk the stairs?** If not, temporarily move a bed to the first floor.

- **Will you be confined to bed?** If so, you may need a hospital bed. Ask your doctor prior to surgery so you can have one at home if you need it.
- **Will your surgery leave you so weak or otherwise limit your mobility (for example hip surgery) that it will make it difficult for you to get around?** If so, you may need a wheelchair or a cane.
- **Is your home large?** Buy a set of two-way walkie-talkies to make communication easier.
- **Will you need home nursing care?** If your family or a friend can not provide it, most communities have home health agencies that provide nursing assistance. Call in advance to find out what is available. Find out whether they employ registered nurses or health assistants. Ask your doctor what level of care she thinks you will need so you can schedule the right level of support. Also check with your insurance company to find out how such care can be covered.

> Slow recovery still gets you well.

Phasing Yourself Back In

Don't expect to resume life as you knew it all at once. Phase back into everything—work, exercise, even your social life. I believe the best plan is to return to any activity on a part-time basis and then gradually build up your time, as tolerated. Strategize how and when you begin, what you begin first, and how to modify prior activities to begin them sooner.

FOR INSTANCE...
A professor I know had major orthopedic surgery and was anxious to get back to his students. He taught mainly small groups of graduate students. Therefore, he planned on beginning his return to work by having the class meet in his home. Thus, he avoided having to travel and could guarantee his comfort.

Similarly, you can make modifications in other areas. For instance, if you want to return to the gym, you may want to do some indoor biking as a low-impact way to begin exercising. If you begin part-time and gradually increase your activity, I believe you are more likely to be successful. Of course, you want to check with your doctor before you begin or increase any activities.

> The best plan is initially to return to any activity on a part-time basis.

A final thought for you to consider, but an important one. **Slow recovery does not mean a poor recovery.** Just because your recovery is not as fast as you expected or hoped doesn't mean it is not going well. Talk to your doctor if you have any concerns. My guess is that she will tell you that everyone recovers at a different rate. Slow recovery still gets you well in the end.

Key Take Home Messages   14

- Healing and recovery take time—probably more than you expect.

- Be assertive in working with your doctor to define realistic expectations.

- Prepare yourself, your home, and your work for your recovery.

- Initially return to an activity on a part-time basis and then gradually build up.

- A slow recovery still gets you well in the end.

COMMUNITY CARE VERSUS UNIVERSITY CARE

Is my community hospital always the best place for me?

When should I go elsewhere for medical care?

Is all community medical care the same?

Can I go right to a university hospital if I have a special need?

Two Kinds of Care

Community care is the medical care that is provided by your primary-care physician, your in-network specialists, and when needed, your local hospital or other medical facilities.

There are unique advantages to having all of your care take place close to home. You have an established partnership with your doctor and the specialists you see regularly. They are close by when you are ill—when your partnership will be of most value. I believe people are most comfortable in a hospital that is familiar. Even if you have never been a patient in the hospital, you most likely have visited it a few times. It feels familiar, a part of your community.

If you are a patient in your local hospital, it is convenient for family and friends to visit. If your stay is prolonged for any length of time, this can be a big advantage because frequent visitors can be a real support for your recovery and a boost to your spirits.

- **Is my community hospital always the best place for me?**
  I would argue that certain medical procedures and surgeries are best done at community hospitals. Community hospitals care for the majority of common illnesses and surgeries. If you are having something like your appendix or your gall bladder removed, your community hospital is well set up to do it. There is a long list of other common surgeries and procedures   that you can feel confident about having in your local hospital. The doctors and nurses at community hospitals treat common conditions on a daily basis. This is their special expertise.

> Doctors and nurses within your community and at community hospitals treat common conditions on a daily basis.

- **When should I go elsewhere for medical care?**
  The term **university care** includes medical facilities that are:
  - Teaching hospitals.
  - Affiliated with medical schools.
  - Specific to a special type of care, such a cancer, heart disease, or pediatric care.

These are hospitals that specialize in caring for the unusual and complicated cases that are often outside the expertise of the community hospital.

In general, you can expect to get better care for any condition if you are in the hands of doctors and nurses who deal with that specific disease on a daily basis. This is the place to be if you have a rare disease, a complex medical condition, or are dealing with a life-threatening disease. A medical facility that performs a large volume of a given surgery or treats a certain illness often is most likely going to offer you the best probability of a good outcome. **For rare diseases, the volume of experience necessary to provide the expertise you desire is frequently hard to find outside of the university hospital.** This is why I believe that for uncommon conditions or for complications of common conditions, the university hospital is often the best choice.

How much of your care needs to take place at a university hospital will vary, depending on your illness. For instance, while breast cancer, in most cases, may be perfectly well cared for at your community hospital, surgery for pancreatic cancer is something you probably want done at the university hospital. When deciding whether you need to be seen at a university hospital, use the same strategy discussed in chapter 3 for picking a surgeon. You or your medical advocate need to ask your doctor how common your condition is, and how often he cares for patients with it. This is an important question, and your doctor should be open to discussing it with you.

15

> For uncommon conditions,
> the university hospital is often
> the best choice.

• Is all community medical care the same?

Every community has different resources. If you live in or near a large city or in a large metropolitan area, it is possible that your local hospital is a university hospital or is the equivalent of one. **Assess your community resources carefully.**

As your own medical advocate, you want to become familiar with the resources in your community. Find out if your community has university-level resources available, and if so, in which specialties. While we always hope we won't need it, knowing in advance where to go for the best care is a big help when illness strikes. When all things are equal, you want to get your care locally, even if you have a rare or complex condition.

I live near Baltimore, where there are a number of specialized medical facilities. In my town of Columbia, though, there is a community cancer center that offers medical oncology for the management of cancer, including chemotherapy. It offers a radiation service that specializes in cancer radiation therapy. This radiation oncology program is staffed by physicians from a local medical school. Therefore, my community has a resource equivalent to a university hospital.

- **Can I go right to a university hospital if I have a special need?**

  The care for any illness almost always begins with your local doctor. It is only after you have a proper diagnosis and possibly a second opinion that you should decide if your condition requires more specialized care. If your problem appears complex to your doctor, talk with him about getting a second opinion from someone at the university hospital where you might want to be treated. For some medical problems, **a second opinion from the university staff may be all you need.**

  For rare or complex conditions, university physicians sometimes create a care plan that can be implemented by your local doctors, if you prefer. If you do this, you may want to check back with your university consulting physician on a regular basis.

  In some instances, a university hospital may have a clinic specializing in your illness where you can be treated on an outpatient basis for ongoing care. Leukemia is a condition in which this approach is applicable. In other instances, you may have to transfer all of your care to a doctor at the university hospital and work with him to manage your illness for both outpatient care and, if necessary, for any hospital care.

Go for What Is Best

As a wise medical advocate, you need to be involved in the decision as to where you receive your care. I believe a candid conversation with your doctor can help you decide what the best setting is for you. Bring the topic up if your doctor doesn't. Driving out-of-town for medical care is rarely appealing to anyone. However, **you have to determine where you will get the best care.** If it is in your community-care system, wonderful. If not, then the medical advocate does what is necessary to get himself the care he deserves!

Key Take Home Messages

- Doctors and nurses at community hospitals are experts at treating common conditions and illnesses.

- University hospitals specialize in caring for unusual and complicated cases.

- You may need only a second opinion from the university hospital staff.

- Know your care options so you can choose the best location to receive the care you deserve.

15

EXPERIMENTAL TREATMENT— IS IT FOR YOU?

Who qualifies for a research protocol?

How do I find out if a research protocol is available for my condition?

What if I don't qualify or the protocol is far away?

What about experimental drugs?

Who pays if I enter a research protocol?

Research Protocols

Modern medicine advances through new developments in medical science, and medical science advances through the success of medical breakthroughs, including experimental treatments.

New surgical techniques, instruments, drugs, and treatments are tested through what we call research protocols — carefully orchestrated research studies that include human subjects. The important distinction is that research protocols are experimental because the therapy being tested is not yet proven to be safe and effective.

Many people are under the impression that protocols are only for life-threatening illnesses such as cancer, but this is not the case. There are also protocols for a myriad of less-severe illnesses.

Research protocols are not for every illness or every patient. **They are usually considered for patients who have illnesses in which standard treatments have failed or for which there is no known cure.**

If you have a medical problem that has not been resolved through standard therapies, it is possible that you may qualify for a research protocol. However, you should not rush to get into one if you have not yet tried all the proven options.

> Remember, experimental treatments are not yet proven to be safe and effective.

- **Who qualifies for a research protocol?**
  Each research protocol has its own set of criteria that carefully defines who will qualify to be in the experimental patient group, how they will be treated, and how success will be measured. The protocol also defines a special Informed Consent that the patient must understand and sign, which explains, among other things, the known benefits and risks. A research committee charged with ensuring that the safety and well-being of the patient is being protected to the best of its ability must approve all of these documents before the experimental treatment can begin.

> Research protocols define
> how experimental treatments
> are implemented.

There are, unfortunately, patients who have severe illnesses for which there are no accepted effective treatments.

AN EXAMPLE...

A woman was diagnosed with an advanced stage of brain cancer for which there was no known effective treatment. She was told there were some treatment options but none had proven to be effective in the stage of her disease. Before she agreed to any treatment, she asked if there were any experimental treatments that might offer her some hope. She found a treatment protocol at Duke University that was targeted at patients with her condition. One of the criteria for admission into the protocol was that she could not have had previous treatment for her disease. She had not, so she qualified and she was admitted to the program.

One of the lessons in this story is that **research protocols have strict entrance requirements.** In this woman's case, had she tried one of the treatment options recommended by her physician, she would not have qualified for the Duke experimental treatment. Therefore, this patient's story provides a second lesson, which is: **Don't rush into treatments that are not likely to help until you have thoroughly searched for options that may offer some degree of hope.**

16

The Down Side

Many, if not most, protocols are structured to compare two modes of treatment: the new experimental approach being tested and another approach, either a treatment already in use or, in the case of non-life-threatening diseases, a placebo (a pill containing no treatment substance). The patients selected for the protocol are divided between the two. **Whether you receive the experimental treatment or the standard treatment (or even** the placebo) is decided randomly. **There is no guarantee that you will be part of the experimental group.** This should all be explained to the patient in detail when the protocol and its related Informed Consent are discussed.

> In most protocols, some of the patients do not receive the drug being tested.

- **How do I find out if a research protocol is available for my condition?**

To find out if a research protocol might work for you, talk with your doctor. First, you want to make sure that you have exhausted all proven approaches. If one treatment fails, don't assume you are in need of an experimental treatment; there may be other proven alternative approaches.

If your doctor says that there are no other options to try, you may want to get a second opinion before exploring experimental treatments. In either case, you want to be satisfied that there are no more proven treatments you can try before you consider a research protocol.

If your doctor does not know of any protocols, then you should definitely go for a second opinion. I suggest you seek one from a specialist at a university hospital, who is most likely to be aware of research protocols being conducted in her specialty. Be sure to ask if there are protocols being conducted at other hospitals. If there is more than one protocol available, explore which is the best for you. **Finding out information about research protocols is one place where the Internet can be of help.** (See chapter 17 for Internet research tips).

Discuss whatever information you gather with your doctor. Ask her to contact any protocol program you are interested in. Though you can contact the center yourself, going through your doctor is often more effective.

> There are multiple resources to find experimental therapies. Let your doctor help you with them.

- **What if I don't qualify or the protocol is far away?**

  One of the problems with medical protocols is that they usually have very strict criteria for who can participate. **Whether you can participate also depends on where the protocol is taking place.** They can take place at a single location or at multiple centers throughout the country. Traveling to take part in a protocol can be a hardship, both physically and financially.

- **What about experimental drugs?**

  If a protocol involves a new use for an existing drug or combination of drugs, your doctor may be able to treat you identically without being a part of the protocol. Talk to her about it. Many cancer research studies, for example, include experiments with new combinations of existing drugs. This is the type of experiment that your doctor may be able to do if you can't take part in the formal protocol. This is also a way to get around your insurance company if it is not willing to cover you as part of an official protocol. If your doctor uses existing drugs in a new combination, the treatment most likely will be covered by your insurance.

  > If you cannot be part of a protocol involving a new use of an existing drug, your doctor may be able to treat you identically to the experimental plan.

  16

- **Who pays if I enter a research protocol?**

  The research sponsor will usually cover all of the direct expenses. For instance, a drug company will cover the cost of the drug. It can vary as to whether or not the sponsor will pay for any required testing. Also, ask if the sponsor will be liable for costs should there be a complication.

  These are answers you need to know before agreeing to enter the protocol. You also need to discuss your plans with your insurance carrier, even if your insurance company will not be paying the expenses.

Key Take Home Messages

- You should investigate a research protocol if you have an illness in which all standard therapies have failed.

- Keep in mind that an experimental treatment means that it is not yet proven to be safe and effective.

- Don't rush into an experimental treatment until you have thoroughly searched for proven options that offer some degree of hope.

- Get your doctor involved in your research and fact-finding efforts. She may be able to offer the same course of treatment, depending on how the study is structured.

INTERNET— FRIEND OR FOE?

What are the pluses of using the Internet?

What are the minuses?

What about chat rooms?

Value Varies for Each of Us

The Internet offers value depending on what you bring to it. People who have a background in science, particularly the health field, know how to evaluate and interpret the wealth of useful information that can be found on the Internet. For those who don't know how to evaluate and interpret it, however, the information is a confusing mass of data because much of it is misleading and contradictory.

If you are going to use the Internet to help you be a better-informed medical advocate, learn how to use health information found on the Internet intelligently or don't use it at all.

- **What are the pluses of using the Internet?**
  The Internet offers a great advantage never before available to the average consumer: an **unbelievable amount of information literally at your fingertips.** The Internet contains medical information from basic explanations about specific diseases to diagnosing and treating specific illnesses to alternative treatments to the cutting edge of medical research, and much more.

- **What are the minuses?**
  There is a vast array of data available on the Internet but **it is not regulated in any way as to its accuracy, source, or even the author.** Anyone can put information on the Internet; it is left to you to figure out what is helpful and what is not. As a result, patients can become completely overwhelmed.

  Depending on what you read, you can be unnecessarily frightened or inappropriately reassured. You could be sent on a wild goose chase pursuing cures that don't exist, or steered away from accepted, proven, effective treatments in order to pursue unproven therapies. Do not underestimate the amount of confusing, contradictory, and even inaccurate information that can be found on the Internet.

  There are significant pluses and minuses to researching health issues on the Internet. You need a strategy if you are going to use the Internet to help you manage your health.

Using Primary Sources

The Internet can be a strong ally in the management of your health as long as you know how to evaluate the credibility of what you find.

There are essential steps in using the Internet to get reliable answers to your medical questions. You need to **be very careful about assessing the articles you read and what advice you take.** Specifically, you should:

- Check the credentials of the person who wrote what you are reading. Make sure it is written by a qualified specialist in the field and/or reviewed by a leading professional authority.
- Check the authenticity of the Web site. Is the site a product of a hospital, medical school, medical journal, or medical professional organization? If so, the information should be credible.

Information that comes directly from a qualified person, place, or journal is considered a primary source and should be the kind of site on which you focus your research. For example, you can feel confident that an article that comes from a professional journal like the *New England Journal of Medicine* has been written by and/or reviewed by leading scholars in the field before it was published in that journal. If you are unsure, or are unfamiliar with the journal or the author, **ask your doctor or a medically trained acquaintance to help you evaluate the source** before you include it in your reading.

17

Companies now exist that will do Internet searches and "evaluate" the material for you. Be cautious about these services unless you are confident that the company's information is trustworthy.

> Don't believe something just because it's on the Internet. Evaluate the credibility of everything you read.

Doing a Search

You need to **be specific about what you are looking for.**
Formulate the questions you have, just like you would before
going to your doctor's office. Then search for those answers.
Simply "browsing" the Internet about an illness is not a good
idea. Don't believe something just because you read it on the
Internet. If you find something that sounds too good to be true,
it probably is.

For example, if you are looking for an experimental treatment
program for your illness, check where the program is taking
place, what medical institution is sponsoring it, and who is
leading the program. It is important to always keep in mind that
the Internet is not supervised.

- **What about chat rooms?**
  Just like Internet Web sites, chat rooms have pluses and
  minuses. On the plus side, you can encounter a group of
  people who are going through similar experiences. You can
  share your thoughts and feelings. You can possibly even find
  leads on where to find proven alternative approaches or
  medical research.

  On the negative side, anyone can access a chat room. You
  can pick up information in a chat room that is entirely
  ineffective and potentially dangerous. You need to weigh what
  you read in a chat room just as you would elsewhere on the
  Internet. Again, take the information you find to your doctor to
  discuss and evaluate it.

Qualified Sites

A safe site is one where you can reasonably expect the information to be accurate and fairly presented. There are a number
of categories of these sites.

United States Government Sites

The federal government offers a number of helpful sites, and
many have links that will take you to additional credible

sources of information. Among these sites are:

- *National Institutes of Health (NIH)*
  www.health.nih.gov
- *Federal Drug Administration (FDA)*
  www.fda.gov
- *Centers for Disease Control and Prevention (CDC)*
  www.cdc.gov
- *Medicare*
  www.medicare.gov

Medical School Home Pages

Most, if not all, of the medical schools in the United States have a Web site. Most of these sites have links to information that is geared to be helpful to patients. You can find them by using the search function on your computer and typing in the name of the medical school.

Scientific and Medical Journals

There are a large number of respected medical journals that publish new research and articles that have undergone peer review by a leading expert or experts in the field. Many of these journals provide Internet abstracts of their research articles. **Understanding these articles requires a degree of medical knowledge.** Don't attempt to interpret the findings on your own. You will be better served if you take the article to your doctor and ask him to review it with you. A sample of the sites available includes:

17

- *New England Journal of Medicine*
  www.nejm.org
- *The Journal of the American Medical Association (JAMA)*
  www.jama.org
- *The Lancet*
  www.thelancet.com
- *Annals of Internal Medicine*
  www.annals.org

Some medical journals charge a fee or require that you subscribe to their site to access their information. You can find information on all medical research for free at **www.pubmed.com**, which is a site maintained by the National Library of Medicine (NLM) and the National Institutes of Health (NIH).

Advocacy Groups

There seems to be a Web site for nearly every disease or syndrome. Many of these are sponsored by large organizations that have the expertise to make certain that the information they put on their sites is accurate and complete. Examples of these groups include, but are not limited to:

- *American Heart Association*
  www.americanheart.org
- *American Cancer Society*
  www.cancer.org
- *American Diabetes Association*
  www.diabetes.org

There are other sites sponsored by small groups of well-meaning people who are doing their best with limited resources. There is always a danger that some of the information on advocacy sites may not have had the thorough scientific review that you want before you accept what it says. You need to be a cautious consumer when you are dealing with these sites and find out about the organizations and the validity of the information presented on their Web sites.

There is another type of advocacy group that supports people who have something in common other than a disease. These can also be good sources for information. An excellent example of this type of group is the American Association of Retired People (**www.aarp.org**), which advocates for the benefit of retirees and other senior citizens.

> There is a large number of Web sites that deal with health care. You must carefully select which ones you put your faith in.

Key Take Home Messages

- There are pluses and minuses to using the Internet to research health issues.

- Evaluate the credibility of anything you read on the Internet.

- Use the Internet to answer specific medical questions rather than generally browsing for information.

- Enter chat rooms with caution.

- There are a large number of Web sites that deal with health care, so you must carefully select which ones you should trust.

17

18

DEALING WITH A CHRONIC ILLNESS

Where can I go for help?

What if my condition means I can no longer work?

What if my child gets a chronic illness?

What if my parent or another adult in my family becomes ill?

How do I deal with someone's traumatic injury?

The Meaning of Chronic

A chronic disease is one that is either permanent or lasts for a duration of at least 3 months. Sometimes it resolves over time, and you return to your former state of health. However, some chronic diseases gradually get worse, or just hang on, neither getting any better nor any worse.

There are also severe chronic diseases with unfortunate consequences; some can lead to a disability that puts a limit on your activities, and some can progress to death. Common among all chronic diseases is that they last a long time, and they tend to change slowly.

TAKE THIS EXAMPLE...

I know three people who all developed multiple sclerosis (MS) at about the same time. For my friend Allen, his symptoms are essentially the same now as they were when he was diagnosed 15 years ago. His condition is stable. He still has MS, but he has not gotten worse.

On the other hand, my friend Rachel has experienced a gradual progression of her disease. She has had increasing pain; decreasing strength, particularly in her legs; and increasing fatigue, among other symptoms. She needs a lot of rest and walks with a cane. She has been on a variety of medicines and has even participated in multiple experimental protocols.

For the third friend, the disease was aggressive. Her symptoms worsened quickly until she became totally bedbound. Sadly, she died of her MS after just a few years.

These three cases illustrate how different the same chronic disease can be from person to person. As a medical advocate, this is important knowledge to have when you or someone you are caring for is diagnosed with a chronic illness.

Every Patient Is Unique

As doctors consider patients and their needs, the fact that every patient is unique is possibly the most important principle they must keep in mind. It is sometimes tempting for doctors to think that they can categorize patients by things like their disease, age, gender, and overall health, and then make a confident prediction on the course the disease will follow. They can't!

The way a disease expresses itself in a given patient—and the way a patient experiences any given disease—is the result of a unique interaction of multiple factors. We have all seen a cold, flu, or virus travel from one family member to the next and affect each person differently. The same is true for more-severe illnesses. You want to be keenly aware of how the disease is affecting you.

FOR INSTANCE...

I have both a relative and a close friend with Crohn's disease, a bowel condition that causes cramping, bloating, and diarrhea, among other symptoms. It can be very painful. My friend Fred has had it for several years, and after his initial problems, he has been largely symptom-free.

My relative Bonnie has also had it for several years, but her experience has been much stormier. She has had to restrict her diet and modify her lifestyle. Despite this, she has had flare-ups so severe that she has had to be hospitalized.

How active a chronic disease is varies among individuals. A disease that remains active throughout a patient's life can significantly affect that person's quality of life.

> Every person's experience
> with a disease is unique.

18

• Where can I go for help?

Being your own medical advocate is crucial if you have a chronic disease. It can make the difference between having the best possible outcome or not. The skills we discussed throughout this book for acute illnesses also apply to chronic illnesses. The only difference is that you have to use these skills for the long haul.

You must plan each step so it will incrementally make your life easier and help keep your illness under control. Another important thing to remember is that you do not have to go through it alone. Whatever your health problem, I am willing to bet that there are a number of potential resources to help you manage your illness.

Working closely with your doctor to manage your illness and utilizing every available option medicine has to offer, however, are not enough. It helps to look for support beyond your medical needs. Some people explore alternative medicine as an adjunct to their medical care. If you are considering going this route, discuss it with your primary care doctor.

For many people, a chronic disease can take an emotional toll. It can lead to depression and impact personal relationships. Diseases that lead to disabilities can also cause financial hardships.

For many chronic illnesses, there are **national nonprofit associations that can help you with these issues.** These groups, like the The National Multiple Sclerosis Society, provide many services. They do more than raise funds to support research. They also are good sources of information on the disease and potential treatments, and they frequently sponsor support groups for patients and family members.

In addition, many of them provide or fund direct services for individual patients. Your doctor can help you identify the reputable associations that deal with your condition. Start by checking the organization's official Web site to get information and links to other relevant sites.

- **What if my condition means I can no longer work?**
  There are many frightening things about a chronic disease, one being the financial hardship that can result from becoming disabled and losing the ability to work and support yourself or your family. Government programs are available to financially help people whose disability has made it impossible for them to work.

  For example, **you may be eligible for Social Security Disability payments and Medicare benefits even if you are not 65 years old.** Check the Social Security Administration for details on eligibility at **www.ssa.gov**.

  Many employers offer disability insurance as part of their employee benefit package or offer it at a reduced rate. If you are offered this option at work and have not signed up for it, I strongly suggest that you do. There are also individual disability policies that you can purchase on your own. Once you are disabled, you will be categorized as having a "pre-existing condition" (see page 222) and you will not be able to obtain disability insurance. The time to investigate this type of coverage is when you are well. It is financial protection for you and your family.

> There are many special resources worth exploring for patients with chronic disabilities.

Rest Is Critical

One of the common problems of any chronic disease is fatigue. The disease itself can cause fatigue as one of its physical symptoms. In addition, most illnesses are emotionally draining which causes both mental and physical fatigue. It goes without saying that doing even the simplest tasks of everyday life can be exhausting if you have a physical disability.

Because your body is fighting an illness, additional rest is often one of the most important things you can do to help prevent the condition from getting worse. Whatever the reason for your fatigue, give into it and get extra rest.

Related to this is often the need to shift some of your former responsibilities to someone else. Fulfilling responsibilities requires energy. The wise medical advocate makes sure she is getting the rest needed to optimize her health.

18

CONSIDER THIS...

I have a friend with multiple sclerosis and a relative with fibromyalgia. It is difficult to overstate how important additional sleep is to these two people. When they talk about fatigue, they describe it as if their "gas tank has suddenly gone dry."

They sometimes say, "I feel like I am too tired to breathe." Everyone gets tired; what they experience is different. They need to go to bed early and sleep late. One

> naps every day. Fortunately, they have the good sense to
> listen to their bodies and get the rest they need.

Resting more than usual is often a challenge for patients because they feel that giving in to their fatigue is giving in to the disease. For some, the pressure of family and work responsibilities make it very difficult to get the extra rest they need. I cannot emphasize enough how important it is for you to consider rest a responsibility, and put it at the top of your priority list.

> Don't underestimate
> the need for rest!

Advice for Caregivers

It is a tragedy when anyone gets a chronic disease, but to me it always seems more tragic when it happens to a child. It is as devastating to the parent as it is to the child. Living with and caring for a person with a chronic illness can drain a family both emotionally and financially.

- **What if my child gets a chronic illness?**
  Resources exist specifically to help the chronically ill child. Examples include Juvenile Diabetes Research Foundation International (**www.jdf.org**), Muscular Dystrophy Association (**www.mdausa.org**), and Juvenile Rheumatoid Arthritis (**www.arthritis.org**). Many offer a wide range of support services. Do not ignore the opportunity to use these organizations' resources. Remember to check with your doctor to identify organizations that can be of help to you.

  There are also special governmental programs for which your child may be eligible. Check with the Social Security Administration Web site about financial and medical insurance programs for disabled children. Be very thorough as you look for possible resources for your child.

- **What if my parent or another adult in my family becomes ill?**

The challenges of being the medical advocate for an adult with a chronic illness require a similar resourcefulness as caring for a child. Most people will encounter this situation with an aging parent or other family member. Many chronic illnesses are common among the aging and you may need assistance outside of the family in dealing with it. **If you are the caretaker of someone with a long-term disability, accept the fact that you can not do it all alone.** As I said before, caregivers need support, too. Make sure that you get adequate breaks from your responsibilities. This is often challenging to arrange, but it is so important for the benefit of you and your loved one.

- **How do I deal with someone's traumatic injury?**

Chronic illnesses usually build gradually, so we can, in some way, prepare for them. Accidents are different because they can change a life without a moment's notice. A good example is a brain injury in which there is little hope of a good outcome. Obviously, the emotional impact can be overwhelming; it impacts the entire family. As the medical advocate for an accident victim, do not overlook the possibility of medical insurance as a source of potential funds to support medical bills, especially if the injury was caused by the negligence of someone else.

Being a medical advocate sometimes can be an awesome responsibility. Keeping your wits about you is important and can make a major difference in the life of someone you love.

18

Key Take Home Messages

- Every patient is unique, and the progression of a chronic illness is not set in stone.

- There are many resources of financial and emotional support available for the chronically ill. Search for them.

- Be prepared! Have disability insurance.

- Having a chronically ill child is a special challenge, and there are special resources available.

- Rest is a critical need for someone with a chronic illness.

- Caregivers can't do it all. Don't hesitate to enlist the help of others.

19

HOME CARE VERSUS NURSING HOME CARE

What kind of care is available?

How do I decide?

Will insurance pay?

Different Levels of Care

There is a time in life when location takes on a bigger significance than ever before—when you or a loved one needs personal-care assistance for a medical problem. Though even a short-term need can create anxiety, it is the long-term need that creates the anguish, especially when, as in most cases, you are making the decision as the medical advocate for a loved one. Taking the next step on behalf of someone who can no longer care for himself is an awesome responsibility. Making the best decision requires an understanding of the options and the impact it will have on the patient and the family.

- **What kind of care is available?**

Personal care assistance can be found through:

- Home Care
- Assisted Living
- Nursing Home Care
- Skilled Nursing Facilities

Home Care

Almost all patients would rather be cared for in their own homes, if possible. **Home allows the patients to be surrounded by familiar sites, sounds, objects, and people.** This can be very comforting. There are many challenges, however, to caring for a chronically ill person at home. The degree of these challenges varies directly with how sick the person is.

> FOR INSTANCE...
> I have an acquaintance Larry, whose wife developed Alzheimer's disease. For many years, he cared for her in his home. At first, he was able to do so unassisted. Eventually, he hired a caregiver who would stay with her during the days, but he would care for her at night. He continued in this fashion until she no longer recognized him or was aware of her surroundings. Then he moved her into a nursing home.

Usually **the most challenging aspect of caring for someone at home is having an adequate number of caregivers.** Too often, families depend on one person to take on the responsibility. If the patient is well oriented, then one person may be able to manage the care, but he will still need at least periodic help. If the patient has some disorientation, then the strain on the caregiver is much greater.

There are many aspects of daily care that may require two people, such as bathing and general bathroom chores. In addition, there may be special care functions that require frequent visits by specialists, such as a nurses or physical therapists.

The toll on the caregivers is both physical and emotional. Care giving is often hard physical work. You must ask yourself if you have the strength to lift and move the patient. It is also very hard emotionally. It is one thing to visit someone in a nursing home and quite another to have to provide intimate nursing care on a day-to-day basis. It often causes you to confront your loved one's disease in ways you did not anticipate. For some individuals or families, this emotional stress is more than they can manage. This is one of the signs that you need an alternative plan.

Another common challenge is the need for special equipment to help make the patient comfortable, such as an adjustable hospital bed. A two-story home can be a challenge in itself for someone who can not manage stairs. The list goes on and on. You need to consider all of them before deciding on home care.

> There are many challenges to caring for a loved one at home.

19

Assisted Living

The simplest type of nursing care to consider is **assisted living.** Assisted living facilities are targeted at older people who do not have major medical illnesses but can no longer safely manage and live alone in their own homes. These facilities are frequently small, in order to provide a more homelike atmosphere. Depending on the facility, residents have their own rooms or apartment-like quarters that they can furnish themselves.

Typically, meals are served in a communal atmosphere

and activities and transportation are provided. If needed, medications are supervised. Assistance with bathing can be provided when needed. Residents usually can retain their own doctors. This is an option that works well for many people, especially for those who are lonely or isolated.

> **FOR INSTANCE...**
>
> About 13 years ago, a relative of mine developed some medical problems and was no longer able to care for herself. Her problems did not need intensive nursing, but they did require supervision, meal preparation, and general support. She lived far from other family members and was unwilling to move. An assisted living facility in her community was a great solution for her. She had her own room with her own furniture. There were always caregivers in the facility to help her when she needed it and to provide general support and meals to her.

Nursing Homes

A **nursing home** provides a level of care that is greater than what is provided at an assisted living facility. A nursing home has more of a hospital look with nurses' stations arranged in corridors. They provide all the services of an assisted living facility plus additional nursing services. If your loved one is very sick and unable to care for himself, assisted living is not an option and the only choice you have will be a nursing home.

> There are some facilities that have both nursing home and assisted living so patients can go back and forth, if necessary.

Some people even have special rehabilitative needs. This is often the case with someone who has had a stroke. Many stroke victims spend a few days in an acute-care hospital and are then transferred to a nursing home for rehabilitation before returning home or entering assisted living.

Skilled Nursing Facilities

A **Skilled nursing facility** is the highest level of care short of a hospital. Here the nurses can manage complex medical conditions. The facilities are frequently used as a transitional facility for patients recovering from hospitalization for a serious illness or surgery. Because of the severity of the medical condition of the patients, more medical supervision takes place than in the other options. Some of these facilities have their own doctors, and some of them work with the patient's own doctor.

• How do I decide?

Picking the right level of care sounds confusing, and frequently it is. Look to the patient's doctor to help you make the decision. Visiting the facilities and talking about the health and needs of your loved one with the staff will usually let you know whether or not the facility is right for him.

Once you understand your options, there are factors you must consider in deciding which choice is best. They include:

- **The patient's medical condition.** This can automatically limit your choice since some options may not be reasonable.
- **The patient's and the family's emotional needs.** This is where guilt often comes into play in a large way. If more than one option is viable, often there are strong positive or negative feelings attached to one or more of the options. For many families, home care in a relative's home is considered a major emotional positive. Some patients, however, feel like they will be an imposition if they receive home care and would prefer to be in some type of nursing facility. Also, the relationships within the family may preclude home care, even if intellectually it seems like the best choice. This aspect of choosing is often the hardest part of the process.
- **The emotional environment of the option.** Certain facilities will seem more or less friendly, more or less tense, or have a definable emotional tone in some other way. The "feeling" in the facility can make it more or less appealing. Go with your instincts.

- **Location.** Sometimes a parent has been living alone a significant distance from other family members. If that parent needs home care or nursing home care, the family may want to move the parent closer to one of the family members.
- **Timing and availability.** If the need for supported care is sudden, the choices are sometimes limited by where a bed is available.
- **Cost.** There may be substantial cost differences among the choices. For instance, if there are family members who are qualified to provide the necessary care at home, this is the most economical option. If it means hiring caregivers to come into the home, then home care might be the most-expensive option.

The wise medical advocate must weigh all these aspects just as they weigh the benefits and risks in so many medical decisions. It is rarely an easy process. However, if you are thoughtful about it and take the time to understand and consider all the issues, you can make the best choice for the patient and his family.

The Financial Factor

If you are considering providing home care, recognize the impact it will have on you. Most likely, it will have emotional, physical, and social costs. Don't underestimate the financial cost; it can mount quickly if you must hire skilled workers to help with care. The hourly cost can vary greatly depending on whether you are talking about a nursing assistant or a registered nurse provided by a nursing agency.

- **Will insurance pay?**
  If the patient has **long-term health insurance,** there may be insurance money to pay for staff to assist you with in-home care. Check the details of the policy. Also, if **Medicare** insures the patient, certain home nursing visits, physical therapy, and hospital beds and other equipment may be covered. It is

important to explore your insurance options; home care can be very expensive without it.

Financing care in a nursing home varies according to the level of the facility. Assisted living is the least expensive, followed by nursing homes, and skilled nursing facilities. **Long-term health insurance** may pay for part or all of any of these facilities. You need to check the patient's individual insurance policy. Long-term health insurance may also pay for some of the expenses of home health care. If the patient has **Medicare,** then there are rules for what is covered.

Typically Medicare covers only skilled nursing facility care. However, **Medicaid** will pay for traditional nursing home care, though it does not pay for assisted living. The glitch is that the patient must pass the financial-need test to qualify for Medicaid. If someone needs nursing home care and does not have the insurance or personal finances to cover it, then sadly the patient must liquidate most of his assets to cover the care. This is called spending down. Once the patient has limited his financial resources to the necessary level, Medicaid will pay for his nursing home care.

There are ways around the spending-down process, but you must follow the rules. For instance, some families have tried to transfer the patient's money to other family members. Medicaid has rules regulating how much money can be transferred, and the timing of it. Make sure that you are in compliance with these rules. Medicaid rules vary from state to state, so you must inquire about them. It's a complex issue, and the full discussion of it is beyond the scope of this book. The Medicare Web site can help you if you need to investigate Medicare or Medicaid more fully. Visit **www.medicare.gov** and go to "search Medicare.gov" and type in "paying for long-term care." Follow the links to find the government programs that cover Medicaid.

19

> The expense of financing either at-home care or nursing home care is a significant issue that families must be prepared to deal with.

Key Take Home Messages

- Investigate the different options before deciding how to provide for a loved one who needs personal care assistance.

- The term "nursing home" can cover a range of personal-care facilities—you need to understand the differences.

- Consider the emotional and financial impact the various care options will have on you as well as your loved one.

- The expense of financing either home care or nursing home care is a significant issue that families must be prepared to deal with.

20

TIMES OF CRISIS

How do I make the right decision?

When Hope Is Gone

For many diseases, there comes a time when it becomes clear that there is no longer a reasonable hope for a cure. If someone is dying, even if death is not imminent, there are many issues that the medical advocate needs to face. The key to making the right decisions is to understand the different approaches in treating the illness when recovery isn't going to happen. Essentially, treatment follows three stages:

- Trying for a cure.
- Palliative care (slowing the progression of the disease).
- Relief of pain and suffering.

One of the hardest decisions you will ever make as a medical advocate for yourself or when entrusted with someone else's care is to **stop trying for a cure and transition to palliative care.** Most people don't want to give up, and they want to hold out for the hope of a miracle, or something close to it. As a medical advocate, however, you need to be a realist and want to be prepared to help avoid needless suffering by the patient. You can recognize this point in time by being aware of the risks and benefits of each treatment decision as it is made.

The reality is that many of the treatments aimed at a cure are aggressive and can create greater discomfort and stress on the patient than those aimed at palliation. Frequently, the patient and/or the family and/or the doctors have a very hard time acknowledging when this point has been reached. However, it is important to recognize this reality so the course of care can be modified.

This does not necessarily mean you give up fighting the disease. Palliative care means you adjust the treatment to try and slow the progress of the disease and prolong the patient's life, but you are not going to continue to put her through treatments with severe side effects that are no longer justified.

An equally difficult decision is knowing **when to stop pushing aggressive palliative care and change the goal to relieve pain and suffering rather than to prolong life.** How do you know? You must pay particular attention to the potential conflict of increasing the quantity of life while decreasing the quality of that life. This changeover is part of the natural progression of a disease. Ask the doctor (and yourself) honestly: *Will the treatment simply prolong life while increasing suffering, rather than prolonging a satisfying life for the patient?*

A variation on this scenario is when the patient has reached a point where the disease itself is causing such suffering that prolonging life is not a caring thing to do. At this point, you have to stop fighting the disease, and you focus all your efforts on limiting any pain or suffering your loved one is experiencing.

> One of the hardest decisions many patients and their loved ones face is when to change the aggressiveness of the medical treatment.

• How do I make the right decision?

There are often no clear-cut lines that signify that you are passing from one phase of the disease to another. You can not overestimate how difficult the decision will be. What often complicates it is a difference in opinion among family members. In the late stages of a disease, there is a tendency for members of the family to want increasing control of the situation.

It is an important form of respect toward the patient that the family **consults with her at each point in the treatment** as long as she is capable of making her own decisions. Autonomy is an important medical ethical principle, and it speaks to respecting the independence of the patient. Late in a disease, **paying attention to your loved one's autonomy is often one of the gifts you can give.**

A GOOD EXAMPLE OF THIS IS...
A friend of mine, Betty, developed breast cancer while she was pregnant. The treatment plan called for surgery, radiation, and chemotherapy. The toxic nature of the chemotherapy would mean that she would lose the baby, so she agreed to the surgery but delayed any further treatment until after the baby was born. She then underwent radiation and chemotherapy.

Unfortunately, she had a recurrence of the disease that, despite treatment, continued to progress. Near the end of

20

her life, she was admitted to the hospital and placed on a respirator. After she got some personal business and papers in order, she began to feel that her pain and inability to breathe without a respirator did not make life worth living.

She requested that the respirator be turned off. The hospital's ethics committee and the family met. It was agreed by all that she was in control of her mental faculties and was making an informed and valid medical decision for herself. She discussed it again with her family, and then the respirator was discontinued. She died peacefully shortly thereafter.

The lesson in this story is that Betty and her family were communicating and her family respected her wishes.

> Paying attention to a loved one's autonomy is one of the gifts you can give.

Hospice Care

Where a patient dies is often an important decision that is made by both the patient and family. No matter where the location, hospice can help with the process and make someone's dying wish possible.

Hospice is a program aimed at providing care in conjunction with physical, emotional, and spiritual support for a terminally ill patient (usually with 6 months or less to live) and her family. Hospice care is most often provided in the patient's home, but in some situations it can be provided in a special hospice facility, a hospital, or a nursing home.

Hospice workers are caring people who are devoted to helping patients and families through the dying process. I would encourage anyone to contact a hospice program when hope of recovery is no longer an option. Many people delay contacting hospice because they see it as giving up. I see it as recognizing the severity of the illness and helping to give someone the best quality of life for whatever time is remaining.

Even before someone might qualify for the full services of hospice, both patient and family may benefit from a consultation with hospice workers.

A Hospice Residence

The same care you can receive with home hospice care can be found in a residential hospice facility. The atmosphere is typically very caring, and the goal is to provide relief from pain and suffering.

FOR EXAMPLE...

Recently, my friend's aunt died after a long bout with lung cancer. Early in her treatment, she visited our local residential hospice facility. She liked it very much and told her family that when the time came, she wished to die there. Her family, with the aid of hospice, did all that was necessary to care for her at home until the family felt the time was right to move her to the facility she had chosen. By the time they moved her, she no longer was able to tell where she was. For the next 10 days, she was well cared for with excellent control of her pain. She died peacefully.

This is an excellent example of how complex the relationships and decisions are during the dying process. What is most important is that the focus remains on caring for the patient and making control of pain and suffering a key priority.

> I cannot speak strongly
> enough about the benefit
> of a hospice program.

20

At Home

Many people want to die at home. Some families find this a wonderful and loving experience, but others find it very stressful. **Everyone involved needs to be honest when this discussion takes place.** If you plan to have your loved one die at home, I strongly encourage you to involve hospice in planning for this care. They can be a tremendous aid in getting the house prepared and provide guidance on how to care for the patient's multiple needs during this time.

> **FOR EXAMPLE...**
> My friend Kate was dying of advanced cancer. All medical treatment options for curing the disease and then for slowing the progression of the disease were exhausted. It was clear that the end was very near. The decision was made to have her die at home.
>
> With the help of hospice, medical support equipment and a hospital bed were set up in her home. A hospice nurse visited daily and was on call 24 hours a day. The staff trained Kate's family how to manage her increasing pain with medication.
>
> Kate began needing more medicine to control her pain, and she began to drift in and out of sleep more often. Despite all this, having Kate home gave her family more time to talk with her and comfort her, and the opportunity to say good-bye. Kate died with her family by her side. Her death was no less sad, but it left the family with the feeling that it was a loving event that honored Kate's wishes.

The Hospital

For a variety of reasons, many, if not most, patients die in the hospital. Some die there because that is where they and their families want them to die. Others die there because events spin out of control and an alternative plan, which might be the desired scenario, never has a chance to play out.

> **FOR EXAMPLE...**
> One evening, my father-in-law, who had had a variety of illnesses over the years, suddenly began throwing up blood. He was rushed to the local hospital, where he received excellent and aggressive care. Initially, his doctors thought they could control the situation. As each decision was made, the doctors told us that they believed they could save him.

> We were aware that he did not want to be kept alive with a respirator or other life-support systems, but before we knew it, he was on a kidney dialysis machine and a respirator. The doctors said that he needed the machines temporarily just to buy some time until the medications kicked in.
>
> Before the night was out, however, his heart failed and he died—in the hospital attached to machines. As a family member who knew him intimately for over 40 years, I can say that each decision made was consistent with our understanding of his wishes, considering his apparent medical condition and prognosis. He died in a relatively short period of time, and we had no reason to think that the machines were functioning as "life support" in the way he had imagined it. Though we wanted to respect his wishes, the circumstances were such that he, unfortunately, died exactly the way he said he did not want his life to end.

This story shows that **it is not always possible to fulfill a person's dying wishes.**

If a person wants all possible efforts made to prolong her life when death is threatening, the hospital is the right place to be. Others may choose the hospital because they have emotional reasons why they do not wish to die at home, or they lack the network of caregivers to support them in their home during the dying process.

Nursing Home

Many people are in nursing homes as they approach the end of their lives. It is important that the nursing home has clear instructions on what the patient and family desire. Often the desire is to let the patient die in the nursing home. If so, you want that to be clear so the patient is not suddenly transferred to an acute-care hospital.

20

> There are a variety of choices for the location of end-of-life care, and it is a highly individual choice.

Emotional and Spiritual Support

Spiritual support for many people means organized religion, but for others, it takes a different form. What is important is to be sensitive to the spiritual side of a dying person and respond in the same way she expresses it. The range of expression is varied. A person may want certain music played or something specific read to her. She may want the holy books of her faith nearby or want to discuss reincarnation.

The list is endless, but you want to be sensitive to your loved one's desires. If someone is trying to express his or her spirituality during this period of life, help them. They will show you how.

How Long?

The doctor will know when death is very close and will be able to tell you at that time. It may not, however, be helpful to ask your doctor to make an estimate earlier on in the disease. Don't be surprised (or annoyed) if the doctor will not give you a direct answer. No one knows with confidence what the precise answer is, and some doctors think it is best to just take things day by day. Not all patients want to know how long they have to live. Look to the patient for your cues on whether or not to pursue this conversation.

Saying Good-Bye

Saying good-bye is often a bittersweet but wonderful process for all involved. Hopefully, by the time your loved one is near death, the relationships between her and her loved ones will feel complete to all. Having the chance to express the love and joy you have found in your relationship is often very healing emotionally for both parties.

I KNOW OF NO FORMULA FOR THIS CONVERSATION
EXCEPT THAT IT SHOULD COME FROM THE HEART...
A dear friend of mine, George, was dying after a 10-year battle with cancer. He knew his death was approaching. He spoke with or wrote letters to many of those who were close to him. He was able to express his love and gratitude, and he made it easier for those he loved and who loved him to do so as well. His death was still a sad event, but the act of being able to say good-bye made it seem that his leaving truly was a part of his life. It somehow made others feel closely connected to him, even though he was gone.

Key Take Home Messages

- There may come a time to stop trying for a cure and to change the care goal to palliative care.

- There may also be a time to stop pushing palliative care and to change the goal to relieving pain and suffering rather than prolonging life.

- Hospice is an excellent resource that offers both medical and emotional support.

- Choosing where you want to die is an important end-of-life decision.

- Saying good-bye can be a comfort to some patients and families.

21

UNDERSTANDING YOUR INSURANCE PLAN

Who's paying for all this health care?

Who decides what plans my employer offers?

How do I decide what type of plan is best for me?

What if I have a child in college or spend my winters in Florida?

How can I get better coverage through Medicare?

What are the Medicare Advantage Plans?

Health Care Is Big Business

More money is spent on health care in the United States per capita than any other nation on earth. The numbers are truly staggering. Health-care costs are growing faster than inflation— 7 percent annually since 2002. In 2003, for example, U.S. health care cost $1.7 trillion—15.3 percent of the gross domestic product! That amounts to an average of $5,670 per person. By the end of this year, the cost is expected to top $2 trillion and cost $6,830 per person.

> Aren't we glad to have
> health insurance!

Health insurance is one of those necessary evils. Without it, a serious illness or injury could wipe us out financially. Having it offers us security—but following all its rules and regulations offers us anxiety, too. Health insurance isn't like other policies that you stick in a drawer and seldom (if ever) have to use. Even if you're in great health, you visit your doctor at least once a year—at least you should—for a physical. As your own medical advocate, you must be sure that you:

- Are always covered and never let your insurance lapse.
- Pick the best plan for you and your dependents.
- Understand your plan completely and thoroughly.

It is not within the scope of this book to describe all the varieties of insurance plans in detail. But I can guide you in selecting your plan and, most important, using it to best benefit your needs. Reading through a bunch of information about insurance is not exciting reading, but stick with me because it is one of the most important tutorials you will be getting in this book.

The High Price of Health

You may be old enough to remember the days when a medical insurance policy came as part of the job. You paid nothing except possibly a modest deductible, and you saw any doctor you wanted.

Those days are gone. Employers, even big employers, are feeling the pinch from rising medical costs and virtually all employees pay part of the share of their health costs through payroll deductions. Here's why: The average annual health insurance premium for a family covered by an employer health plan is around $11,000, and more than $4,000 for an individual. You, the employee, are paying a significant portion of that coverage. At last count, the average employee out-of-pocket share for family coverage was about 25 percent of the employer's health-insurance premium—just over $2,600 per year—and the average individual employee out-of-pocket share is about 15 percent—around $560 per year.

What about the Uninsured?

With numbers like these, it is no wonder that we have so many uninsured people in this country. An estimated 15 percent of Americans (46 million people) do not have medical insurance. This includes the unemployed, low-and middle-income workers who can't afford the employee out-of-pocket share for health insurance provided at work, or those who work for a small business that can't afford to offer health care as a benefit to its employees. The court records are filled with the names of uninsured families that have faced financial ruin over the medical bills of someone who was ill or injured.

If you've ever wondered why emergency rooms are always so full, it is because it is a place people can go for medical assistance when they don't have any insurance. The hospitals treat them, and the expense of their care is eventually spread to the insured through a raise in insurance premiums. **This "free" treatment is taking place in the most expensive outpatient care setting—it is one economic wrong causing another.**

- **Who's paying for all this health care?**
Health care in the United States is funded by a combination of private and public insurance plans. To be a successful health-

care advocate, you need to understand the basics of these programs. Roughly 45 percent is paid through public programs, 41 percent from commercial insurance programs, and about 14 percent ($238 billion) is out-of-pocket spending by individuals.

When I say public programs, I am talking about Medicare, Medicaid, and public programs offered on state and local levels. If you are an able-bodied worker under the age of 65, you probably don't qualify for a penny of these public funds. I know all this is of little comfort, especially if you are among the people who are in a job just to have health coverage. It comes down to the reality that everyone needs some type of health insurance, because the risk of financial ruin without it is too great.

Your Choices: Know the Difference

First and foremost, you should **understand the types of insurance that are available.** There are myriad options in a variety of plans available for individual buyers and through employers—far too many to get into in this book. Essentially, most fall under one of three categories.

Indemnity Fee-for-Service

Indemnity Fee-for-Service once was the most popular because it offers the greatest flexibility of choices in terms of doctors and facilities. It is also the greatest cost to the employee (both in terms of premiums and co-pays), which is why it is rapidly disappearing.

It is called Indemnity Fee-for-Service because it indemnifies (protects) you against medical costs. Fee-for-service means the doctor is paid on some type of fee schedule, usually based on rates established by the insurance company, for each service he provides you.

In addition to your monthly premium, you are also responsible for **deductibles and co-pays.** Most indemnity insurance policies do not start paying for your health care until you satisfy your yearly deductible, a pre-set out-of-pocket expense. Once you have paid the deductible, the insurance pays its share of your medical bills. **The amount of the deductible varies with the**

policy, but it is often in the range of $250 per person and $500 per family. If you are considering indemnity insurance, you need to know this number!

Even after the deductible is met, an indemnity policy typically only pays a portion of your remaining medical bills, and you pay the rest out-of-pocket. For example, insurance might pay 80 percent and you pay an out-of-pocket **co-pay** of 20 percent. The percentage varies among policies, so make sure you understand how much you are liable to pay. If you end up in the hospital, for example, your 20 percent can added up to a lot of money.

Managed Care (HMO)

Most people think of **Managed Care** as a Health Maintenance Organization, commonly called an HMO. They are the most tightly controlled type of insurance policy. If you belong to an HMO, you pay a monthly premium and have your care managed by a Primary Care Provider (PCP). A PCP is usually a family practitioner, an internist, or a pediatrician. (Currently in California, an acupuncturist can also be a PCP). Some insurance plans also define the obstetrician/gynecologist (OB/GYN) as a primary care provider.

Usually an HMO will not pay for you to see a specialist, such as a dermatologist or cardiologist, without a referral from your PCP. Some policies require a pre-authorization, that is prior approval from the insurance company, before it will allow certain tests or even hospitalization. You want to know this up front and understand the rules, because you will be required to follow them. If you don't, you could get stuck with a shocking medical bill because you failed to get the necessary approvals in advance.

Under a managed-care system, you generally must see only doctors who participate with the HMO. The panel of doctors contracted by the HMO is known as the "network." These are doctors who have agreed to the management program and fee schedule of the HMO. For some very specialized care, you may be sent out-of-network, but this generally requires pre-approval by the HMO. In addition to your monthly premium, you usually have a flat co-pay for each doctor's visit. This is usually about $10 to see your PCP. Frequently, the co-pay for a visit to a specialist or the emergency room is more, around

21

$25. If you go out-of-network without pre-approval, your care may not be covered at all. You do not want to make this mistake. If you belong to an HMO and want to see an out-of network doctor, make sure you have an approved referral in writing first!

The advantages of the HMO include lower premiums and out-of-pocket expenses. It is a particularly good plan for young families with children who require frequent visits to the doctor. The disadvantage for some patients is the limited choice of doctors in the network and the degree of management the PCP has over your care. For example, if you want to see a specialist, you must first talk to or see your PCP. Only with his agreement can you go to the specialist. Also, the referral networks for HMOs are often smaller than other types of health insurance, so your choices are more limited.

Preferred Provider Organization (PPO)

A **Preferred Provider Organization**, or PPO, is somewhat of a blend between Indemnity Fee-for-Service and an HMO. PPOs are **currently the most popular form of insurance plan**. In a PPO, you also have a panel of doctors—a network—that the insurance company prefers you to use. You usually pay a fixed co-pay for each visit within the network similar or higher in amount to an HMO. There may or may not be a requirement for you to select a PCP. There are typically no referrals required for you to see a specialist.

PPOs have an advantage over an HMO because they allow you to see a doctor outside the network. Each visit to an out-of-network doctor will cost more than a visit to an in-network doctor, but your insurance will honor the bill. Typically, when you go outside the network, the PPO financially operates like an indemnity policy. This means that you will have to meet a deductible before you receive any benefit, and after the deductible is met, your co-pay is a percentage of the insurance company's approved fee—not what the doctor may charge.

These differences in payment create **significant financial incentives to stay in the network.** For instance, it might cost you only a $25 co-pay to see a dermatologist in-network, but you might have to pay the entire cost of the care to go out-of-network if you haven't met your deductible. Details on co-pays, deductibles, and networks vary from one PPO to another. You need to understand how your plan works!

- **Who decides what plans my employer offers?**
  Your employer chooses the insurance company and decides which of the insurance company's plan or plans are offered. The employer can even alter provisions of the plans, such as the amount of the co-pay and deductible. In addition, many insurance companies will let an employer modify the medical benefits offered within the plan. Therefore, the challenge to you as the employee is to pick the plan that will work best for you. If you are not satisfied with any of the plans offered, work with your employer to see if the options can be improved.

> There are many types of private health plans—not every plan is for everyone. You need to understand yours.

- **How do I decide what type of plan is best for me?**
  This is a very individual choice. There are some generalities, but you need to decide for yourself.

In general, **Indemnity Fee-for-Service** plans are:
- More expensive.
- Offer the most freedom of choice.
- Often good for older patients who may want specific doctors for their medical conditions.

In general, **HMOs** are:
- Less expensive.
- Usually very good for routine care.
- Good for families with children because they usually include more preventive-care benefits and a low co-pay for office visits.
- Tightly controlled, meaning you'll need to get a referral from you primary-care physician for specialty care.

21

In general, **PPOs** are:

- Less expensive than indemnity fee-for-service but more expensive than HMOs.
- Offer greater freedom of choice than HMOs.

As a medical advocate, you need to assess the pluses and minuses of the insurance options as they fit your current needs. Over the course of your lifetime, your choice will change as your needs change.

A GOOD EXAMPLE OF THIS PROCESS IS...

My wife and I belong to a PPO. As empty-nesters, we enjoy the greater freedom of choice and the ability to see a specialist without being referred. Our primary concern is that our PPO network includes our primary-care physicians, who have known us for a long time and give us guidance on our overall care. The network also includes nearly all the other physicians we would want to use, should the need arise.

Our three grown children have made their individual choices based on their own needs. My son, Greg, is married and has two small children. He has chosen an HMO because he prefers the lower overall cost. He does find the more-restrictive network a problem at times, as he may have to drive farther for an x-ray, for instance, because the facility nearest to him is outside the network.

My oldest daughter, Kim, who is married and has three children, belongs to what the insurance company calls an open-access HMO. This is slightly more expensive than a traditional HMO. It still has the referral requirements of an HMO, but the network is much bigger. Her son has had surgery in the past, and she wants the greater freedom of choice the open-access HMO offers her.

Amy, our youngest child, is not married and has no children. Her career involves extensive travel within the United States, so she belongs to a PPO with a national network. Her PPO does not require her to check in with a PCP, and she finds this very helpful. She can be almost anywhere in the country and find in-network primary-care doctors or specialists.

As you can see, there are some generalities that will help you in selecting your insurance. The specifics involve your lifestyle. These are the questions you should ask yourself:

- How critical is the expense of my health care?
- How critical is the freedom to access the greatest number of doctors and facilities for my health care?
- Are the doctors I see or may want to see in the network?
- Do I have special health care needs that I want to be sure are covered by this health-care plan?

Consider Your Lifestyle

When you consider your plan you have to consider your life style. If you rarely are far from home, an HMO might work well for you. **If you have a job that requires you to travel many days a week or a month than an HMO might be a poor choice for you.** An Indemnity Fee-for-Service plan or a PPO might work well for you in this scenario.

- **What if I have a child in college or spend my winters in Florida?**

  An HMO that has no away-from-home benefits other than emergency care is not for you. However, some insurance plans, even **some HMO's, have provisions to deal with you or a member of your family living part of the year out of the area.** Some health plans have either national networks or alliances with related plans in other areas or other states. You need to look into this as a needed option.

  The insurance needs of a child in college can be managed much the same as for any family member who spends significant time away from home. Another option for an out-of-town student is to **find out if the college has a health plan** that will cover him while he is at school. Most schools have some form of health plan available. If so, make sure to study the details of the plan. You want to know how expensive it is, and what its benefit package covers.

  Some in-school policies are very limiting and only cover acute

21

problems, meaning your child will be covered if he gets sick or injured and needs immediate attention. This is fine for the emergency, but it is not the whole picture. For instance, if your child injures his knee, the emergency care will be covered, but if he needs surgery or physical therapy, it may not be covered by the school insurance. If your family policy is an HMO that requires him to use in-network providers for physical therapy, then it may mean that your son could miss a semester at school.

In my role as an insurance executive, I have seen such a scenario played out many times. It is not a happy scene. Look for a school policy with more complete benefits and pick a family plan that covers someone while away from home.

> Look at the specifics of the plan and compare them to your own health needs and the needs of others in your family.

Now You're on Medicare!

Medicare is the largest insurance plan in the country, with some 40 million enrollees. As with private plans, not all Medicare is the same. One of the difficulties of retirement, some will say, is trying to figure out your Medicare options.

There are two major types of Medicare plans:
- Original Medicare Plan
- Medicare Advantage Plans (formerly called Medicare+Choice or Medicare Part C)

The Original Medicare Plan has two medical-care components:
- Medicare Part A
- Medicare Part B

You are eligible for Original Medicare if you are:
- A U.S. citizen or permanent resident of the United States.
- Age 65 or older.

- You or your spouse have worked for at least 10 years in Medicare-covered employment (you paid Medicare taxes).

Medicare Part A is free, and it is called the hospital component. It covers hospitalization, skilled nursing facilities, hospice care, and some home health care. **Medicare Part B** requires you pay a premium, and it is called the doctor's component. It covers the bills for doctors' services as well as for some other health-provider services, like outpatient hospital care, some physical therapy and occupational therapy, and some home health care. As of 2006, the cost to most people for part B is $88 per month, plus an annual deductible of $110. However, this can vary.

Medicare Part D is the Medicare drug benefit and is discussed in chapter 23.

If you are a U.S. citizen or a lawfully admitted alien who has lived in the United States for at least 5 years, you can also get Medicare benefits, even if you do not meet the employment requirement. However, you will have to pay a premium for your Part A coverage as well as the usual premium for Part B.

- **How can I get better coverage through Medicare?**
  There are some aspects of your medical care that the Original Medicare Plan Part A and Part B do not cover, like co-insurance, co-payments, and deductibles, some of which can be **significant out-of-pocket expenses.** To offset the costs, you can buy insurance for many of these gaps through a **Supplemental or Medigap Plan** that you can obtain through a private insurer. In addition, a Medigap policy can provide you with additional benefits beyond the basic Medicare benefit package, such as foreign travel emergency care or at-home recovery care. There are 12 standard Medigap insurance plans, known by the initials "A" through "L", each with its own set of benefits. Decide what benefit package you want, then check the price, as the same standard benefit package can vary from one insurer to another.

21

- **What are the Medicare Advantage Plans?**
  Medicare also offers another group of options called Medicare Advantage Plans that cost more out-of-pocket but offer more services than you would get through a Medigap plan. It is also

purchased from a private insurer. You receive a private insurance card from the plan, and you use it to pay for the care you receive.

If you decide to join a Medicare Advantage Plan, you still need to join Medicare Part A and Part B, but these plans may offer additional benefits above the Original Medicare Plan. Your out-of-pocket expenses vary with the plan.

There are four types of plans:
- Medicare Managed Care plans
- Medicare Preferred Provider Organization plans (PPOs)
- Medicare Private Fee-for-Service plans
- Medicare Special Needs plans

The first three types are similar to commercial insurance counterparts. The **Medicare Managed Care** plans are like HMOs: your care is managed by a PCP, you need referrals to specialists, and you are limited to a network of doctors in return for lower out-of-pocket expenses. The **Medicare PPOs** offer more freedom than an HMO and the opportunity to go out of network, but you accept the possibility of greater out-of-pocket expenses. The **Medicare Private Fee-for-Service** plans are like private indemnity policies—you accept higher expenses for more freedom of choice. The **Medicare Special Needs** plans are focused on a group of patients with a common medical need. For instance, there are Special Needs plans that focus on nursing home patients and diabetic patients.

For both Medigap and Medicare Advantage plans, you pay a monthly premium to the insurance company, and Medicare pays a monthly premium to the insurance company on your behalf in return for the insurance plan providing your health-care insurance. The plan will then pay for your medical care according to the provisions of the plan.

> There are Medicare options that vary in their benefits, expenses, and freedom of choice. Be a wise medical advocate and find the one that is best for you.

Key Take Home Messages

- Understand the differences in insurance plan options and choose the one that best meets your current needs.

- The "free" part of Medicare does not cover all of your medical needs. Study the options and pick the best one that you can afford.

- There are gaps in the Medicare coverage. You want to fill them.

22

NAVIGATING YOUR INSURANCE POLICY

Must I read the entire booklet?

What do I do if my employer changes insurance plans?

What should I do if I have a pre-existing condition?

Does health insurance cover all conditions that are not pre-existing?

Why do doctors keep changing what insurances they accept or what networks they are in?

How does the way doctors get paid impact my relationship with my doctor?

Who pays when the doctor and insurance company don't agree?

What should I do if I receive a bill in error?

Your Policy Is a Contract

It is my experience both in medicine and health insurance that most people do not really read, and therefore do not understand, their insurance policies—until they have a problem. Oftentimes, by then it is too late. There's a saying "The devil is in the details," and it is particularly true when it comes to your health insurance policy.

> A health insurance policy is a contract. You need to know as much as possible about the details before you sign up.

Your medical insurance policy is really a contract between you and the insurance company. This is an important fact that you should not overlook. It is not a contract between you and your employer. The contract comes to you in the form of the **benefit booklet that is sent to you by the insurance company after you sign up for the insurance with your employer or insurance agent.** The only way you'll know exactly what you've signed up for is to read your plan booklet. It is not enough to read only the summary.

• Must I read the entire booklet?

Even if you've done your advance homework to select a plan as I suggested in chapter 21, you could get caught by surprise if you are not familiar with, as they say, the fine print. Plans are generally presented to enrollees in the broad terms that affect a majority of the policyholders. It is possible that information on one or more concerns that affect you can be found only by reading all the fine print.

The smart medical advocate will investigate all her concerns ahead of time. You can do this by talking to your insurance agent or your company's human resources department.

> You want to consider your individual and family's health needs when picking a benefits package.

Know Your Benefits

Before signing up for your policy, you want to make sure that you are getting the benefits that matter to you the most. Predict as best you can what you might need over the coming year— physical therapy, home care, specialty care, medications. Does your policy cover you when you go outside the local network of providers? Does it offer the alternative therapies that you are interested in? All these things are important because they will impact the management and quality of your health care.

- **What do I do if my employer changes insurance plans?**
  You get your plan as close as it can get to what you want, then find out that your company is changing your plan and you must go through the aggravation all over again! You are not alone. This is an increasingly common employee complaint and another unfortunate reality of what's wrong with the current medical system. As insurance premiums continue to rise, employers continue to shop around their health insurance for the best rates.

  It is becoming more and more common for employers to price-hunt and change insurance plans every 1 to 3 years. If the low bidder keeps changing, so does your insurance carrier. Sometimes your employer will change plans within the same insurance company, and sometimes your employer will change insurance companies. In either case, it means that if your doctor is not part of the new plan, you will have to change doctors.

  If you are lucky, your company offers more than one insurance plan and you will at least have options from which to choose. But there are many companies that offer only one plan.

  If this happens where you work, find out why. **It is possible that the new policy is cheaper to your employer because the benefit package is not as complete as the former policy.** It could also mean higher co-pays for you. Your best bet is first to carefully compare the benefits of the old plan to the new one. If you have issues, take them to your employer. In my experience with employers, I have seen them respond to this type of input from their employees. Your employer will not be able to change the plan offered for this year, but it can change it for future years. Remember, you are in the health-insurance game for the

22

long run. Even if you can't optimize this year, it is worth talking to your employer about future years.

> Any time your insurance company changes, check the new benefit package to see if your doctor is in the new network.

Pre-Existing Conditions

Insurance is a business, and businesses exist to make money. Insurance companies make money by collecting more in premiums than they pay out in claims. It's kind of like Atlantic City. They gamble that when you buy a policy, you won't need to use it. So, if a person with a bad back or a bad heart wants to buy insurance, they see it as a bad bet—and they don't want to play. They call this a **pre-existing condition,** and it can create a big problem if you are trying to buy insurance.

If you or anyone in your family has a pre-existing condition, you want to **make sure that there is no waiting time or permanent exclusion in your policy for treating a pre-existing condition.** This may not be an issue if you are getting your insurance through your employer, though the size of the company you work for can be a factor. **For companies with more than 200 employees,** insurance is offered as a group policy, and pre-existing conditions are not a barrier to joining the plan.

At the other extreme, if you need to buy an **individual policy** for yourself or your family, you may not be able to obtain insurance at all if someone has a pre-existing condition. Or, you may get a policy that will exclude coverage of the condition for a period of months or the life of the policy.

For companies with 50 or less employees, it is possible that one employee's pre-existing condition could result in overall higher premiums for everyone in the plan, or the person could be disqualified from the plan. **For companies between 50 and 200 employees,** the issue could go in either direction. You need to talk to your employer.

- **What should I do if I have a pre-existing condition?**

  If you have a pre-existing condition and are having trouble getting insurance, you may have some options. Some states require certain insurers to have open-enrollment periods where they will accept anyone who applies, regardless of their health status. **There are often limited time periods each year when you can enroll.** If this applies to your family, you need to evaluate these programs very carefully. Also, the benefit package may not be as comprehensive as you would like. Unfortunately for some people, this is the only option available to obtain health insurance.

- **Does health insurance cover all conditions that are not pre-existing?**

  I don't know of **a single medical insurance plan that covers all conditions.** Cosmetic surgery is one example. Many plans, however, will cover plastic surgery to correct some injuries and certain birth defects. In addition, different insurance policies may have specific exclusions for other conditions or procedures, such as **fertility treatments.** Some policies may only cover certain procedures, like diagnosing the cause of the infertility, but not cover some or all of the treatments. If you have a special need, you need to talk to the insurance company to find out the details of coverage for that condition. Then talk to your doctor about what her recommendation is for your medical care. In chapter 24, you'll learn strategies you can use to work with your insurance company when they tell you no.

The Problem with Networks

Before the days of out-of-control medical costs, you could pretty much count on your employer to offer a good family medical plan and stay with it. You had the security of having the same benefits and seeing the same doctor year after year. Not so anymore.

When you are changing plans, you want an insurance policy that includes your current doctor or doctors. You can check this out before you sign up by looking at the list of providers the insurance company hands out or by going to the insurance

22

company's Web site. From my experience as an insurance company executive, I can tell you that the insurance companies work hard to make these books and their Web sites accurate. However, as a practicing physician and the manager of a medical group, I can tell you there are many errors in these sources. I strongly advise that you **call all your doctors' offices to verify that they are participating in the plan that you are considering.**

With the way networks work these days, I have to warn you that there may be times when you will be unable to find a plan that includes all the doctors you want. This raises some difficult choices for the family.

> Be sure that the doctors you go to participate in the plan you are choosing. If they don't, carefully consider which plan offers the network that is the best for you.

- **Why do doctors keep changing what insurances they accept or what networks they are in?**

Doctors would like to be available to see all patients, no matter what the patient's payment method. However, in the current medical system, different insurance plans and networks pay doctors different amounts for the same office visits or procedures. So one thing doctors consider when joining a network is how much they will be reimbursed. Another consideration is how many patients the office will get by joining the plan. If the plan can bring a large volume of patients, they may accept a lower fee per procedure in exchange for the opportunity to do more procedures.

These economic considerations of dollars per unit of work and volume of units, unfortunately, have forced doctors to run their practices more like a business. If a doctor gets a lower fee, she must see more patients in the same amount of time in order to maintain her income. As the insurance companies work to pay less per encounter, and doctors work to keep their incomes from dropping, **the patient gets caught in the middle**. This is one of the drivers that is making the medical-care system such a mess—and it is frustrating for both patients and doctors.

The patient is unhappy because she ends up with less time with the doctor. If the doctor concludes that she is not getting an adequate income by being part of the network, she can drop out or change networks. This usually happens when a doctor sees that she will get an adequate number of patients by joining a better-paying network. That could leave you, the patient, looking for a new doctor.

These are purely economic considerations and neglect the impact on the individual patient. If the patient is lucky, she will have access to her doctor's new network. Keep in mind that most employees can usually only change insurance plans once a year. If your doctor drops out of a network part way through your insurance year, you may have to wait many months before you have the option of choosing an alternative insurance plan that your doctor participates in.

If you need to see a doctor in the meantime, you'll have to pick a new one. Call the doctors you are considering to make sure they are accepting new patients. Sometimes, a doctor's practice gets so busy that she temporarily stops taking new patients, no matter what insurance plan you have.

> The economic factors that are causing doctors to change networks result in behavior that is unsatisfactory and frustrating for both patients and doctors.

How Doctors Get Paid

When I started my medical practice 30-some years ago, commercial insurance companies still reimbursed doctors based on what was called the **UCR (Usual, Customary, and Reasonable) System**. This system was based on two criteria: The amounts an individual doctor typically charged for a given visit, test, or procedure, and the amount other doctors in the same community charged. The insurance company would then determine if the charge was reasonable.

Basically, the insurance companies combined these factors and paid the doctor what she charged for a given procedure as long as it was within the customary charges of her medical community. The doctors liked this system because if a doctor raised her charges, usually within about a year, she would also receive an increase in her reimbursement from insurance companies. This system, unfortunately, created an incentive to raise rates.

Medicare, which began in 1965, threw a monkey wrench in the UCR system. During the early years, Medicare developed a reimbursement system with a set fee schedule based on what it calls **RVUs (Relative Value Units).** This system defined that certain procedures were worth more than others and set a given amount that a doctor would get paid for each procedure. Medicare paid what their fee schedule stated and no more. The critical change was that the doctor's reimbursement was no longer tied to her charges, but rather to a fee schedule created by a third party.

The private insurance carriers eventually followed suit and gradually changed to an RVU-based system. Today, most insurance reimbursement is based on pre-set fee schedules, rather than the charges set by the doctor.

As total medical-care costs rose in the 1990s and early 2000s, one of the ways insurance companies attempted to control costs was to either lower their fee schedules, freeze them, or, if they raised them, raise them at a lower rate than inflation. So, in effect, as medical costs go up, doctors' salaries come down. **If they want to keep their salaries stable, doctors have to see more patients and do more procedures.**

> Doctors do not control what they get reimbursed by public and private insurance companies. The only people who pay the doctor's full charges are self-paying patients.

- **How does the way doctors get paid impact my relationship with my doctor?**
The current medical-care system has left doctors with only a few choices—none of which they like. If they continue to work as hard as they've always worked, total income goes down.

What it means is that a doctor who works the same number of hours and sees the same number of patients is actually making less money than she was 15 years ago. If a doctor wants a raise, she has to work longer hours. This is because instead of raising the fee schedules with inflation, the public and private insurers have tried to control the rise in health-care costs by paying the doctors less.

Patients feel the impact of this and commonly complain that they encounter shorter office visits, double-booking, doctors rushing out of the exam room, and doctors being less willing to spend time discussing concerns, especially those that are not specifically related to the reason for which the patient is being seen. These are some of the things that probably came to mind when I declared at the beginning of this book that the medical-care system is a mess.

The net effect has been unhappy patients and unhappy doctors. This leads to a breakdown in the patient/doctor relationship, **and it is why you need to be your own medical advocate or an advocate for your family. You can have the relationship and time with your doctor that you deserve. Unfortunately, it is not going to happen automatically.**

> The changes in the way physicians are reimbursed by insurance companies and Medicare has had a negative impact on patient/doctor relationships.

• Who pays when the doctor and insurance company don't agree?

You do! This is something you need to fully understand. **The amount the insurance company pays is usually calculated from the insurance company fee schedule and not from what the doctor charges.** Unfortunately, doctors and insurance companies don't always agree on fees. This means that if the doctor charges $150 for a procedure, but the insurance company fee schedule allows $100 for that procedure, the insurance company will only pay 80 percent, or $80. This is not because the doctor overcharges. It is because the insurance company pre-determines what it is willing to pay a doctor for each type of visit or to perform each kind of procedure.

It means that after you pay the $20 co-pay, there is a balance of $50 that your doctor charged that is not yet paid. If your doctor charges you for that balance, it is called **balance billing.** Whether she charges you depends on what the doctor's contract is with the insurance company. Blue Cross/Blue Shield plans, for instance, offer contracts that prevent in-network doctors from balance billing. However, out-of-network doctors can balance bill you. Find out what your insurance company's policy is on balance billing. It doesn't seem fair, but that is the way it works.

Co-pays and fee schedules vary from company to company and policy to policy, and contracts can vary between insurance companies and doctors. Therefore, for your own protection, you have to be familiar with the "fine print" of your policy, how its payment mechanism works, and what your doctor's relationship is with your insurance company. For example, can she balance bill? The wise health-care advocate finds out what the financial expectations of a doctor, hospital, or other facility are before agreeing to their care.

Know what you are signing up for. Every time you use the health-care system, you sign a payment form that says you agree to pay all expenses if your insurance company does not. **Don't sign the form as the responsible party if you don't under-stand what you are committing to!**

Ask for the details in advance. If necessary, call your insurance company. Some people think they can agree to pay, and if the bill is too high, they won't have to pay it. It is true that some health-care providers will not come after you if you don't pay the full bill, but some will! It is much better to sort things out in advance.

Those Bills!

With all the paper work that is involved in medical insurance plans, it is no surprise that things get all fouled up. It can happen even if you are doing everything right—I know this from personal experience.

AS I SHARED EARLIER...

I am a patient being followed closely by my team of doctors for an as-yet-undiagnosed mass in my head. In my multiple prior roles in medicine and medical insurance, I have learned about the need for referrals, pre-authorizations, and taking along the necessary forms when I have a test or procedure. I know the rules, and I follow them carefully. Nonetheless, at one point in my treatment, I began receiving bills from the hospital where I had my MRIs. I was being billed personally because my insurance plan hadn't paid.

The first time it happened, I spoke to a case manager and it was taken care of—I never heard another word about it. It happened a second time, so again I pursued it. The case manager said that this should not be happening since everything was submitted properly. She decided to add a special pre-authorization number in "the system" to ensure the billings would stop.

I was given the name of yet another case manager who was in charge of implementing this plan. I was supposed to call back if it happened again. It did. I called the case manager and faxed in all my paperwork, as instructed. She told me not to worry. I didn't, until I got a notice from the hospital that I had been referred to a collection agency. Needless to say, I was not a happy camper at this point. I contacted the case management again...

You get the picture. Between the size of the insurance companies and the hospitals and the volume of patients and paperwork they manage, problems do occur. But if you have your paperwork, and your doctor's office or the insurance company did the billing wrong, the error will be corrected. But you have to be your own advocate to ensure this.

- **What should I do if I receive a bill in error?**
  If you get bills from doctors or hospitals that you think your insurance company should have paid, do not ignore the bills. Either call the doctor or hospital and ask why you got a bill, or call your insurance company and find out why you are being billed directly. Although it is possible it will all get straightened

22

out on its own, it is also possible that you will end up, like I did, with a collection agency on your case. Don't let it happen.

Key Take Home Messages

- A health-insurance policy is a contract. Read it word-for-word.

- Know your benefits package, including which doctors participate in each different plan, before signing up.

- Get all the details and find out what it means to you when your employer changes insurance plans.

- Never ignore an incorrect bill.

PHARMACY AID—FINDING RELIEF FROM RISING HEALTH COSTS

Why should I use one pharmacy?

How does a drug get on the formulary?

How do generic drugs differ from brand-name drugs?

How do I get my drugs added to the formulary?

What does it mean to me if I have Original Medicare with a Medigap policy?

What if I have a Medicare Advantage Plan?

How does this apply if I am a retiree with a health insurance benefit from my former employer?

What do I do if I am going on vacation and will run out of a medicine?

Are there other ways to save money on my medicines?

Know Your Pharmacist

Without a doubt, drug plans are a major hot button when it comes to costs—for both insurance companies and consumers. Americans fill an estimated **3 billion prescriptions** annually, according to the most recent statistics. **This averages to a little over 10 prescriptions per person per year.** That's a lot of medication! And this doesn't count over-the-counter medications, which are not covered by insurance.

Every month, about 43 percent of Americans receive at least one prescription, and well over half of the people who leave a doctor's office walk out with an average of 2.3 prescriptions. Most significant, however, is that many patients are receiving prescriptions from more than one doctor. This is why you need to pay close attention to what you are taking and why **your pharmacist needs to be part of your health team.**

> On average, there are over
> 10 prescriptions per person
> per year filled.

- **Why should I use one pharmacy?**
  As part of your team, your pharmacist can do much more for you than fill your prescriptions. He can:

  - Help you understand the drugs you are taking.
  - Advise you about the risks.
  - Caution you about the interaction between drugs when you are taking more than one.
  - Help you understand your insurance drug benefit.

Given the large number of prescription drugs available, you will, over time, end up needing a variety of prescription drugs for short-term and sometimes long-term illnesses or health problems. All medications have a healing effect and potential side effects. In addition, **many drugs interact with each other in ways you can not predict.** This is why you should have all your prescriptions filled at the same pharmacy or pharmacy chain.

Most pharmacies keep all their prescription files in the

computer. Pharmacies can keep track of all the medicines you are taking that were purchased from any pharmacy in its chain. **The computer programs can check each new medicine against the others you are taking to look for negative interactions.** This is important because two drugs might be very good for you individually, but taken together, they could interact and cause you significant harm.

If you have more than one doctor in your health-care team, they may not be aware of all of the medications other doctors have prescribed for you. By having all of your prescriptions filled at the same pharmacy, you have a very good chance that the pharmacy computer will spot a potential problem and alert the pharmacist. He can then work with you and your doctors to decide what is the best combination for you. You can help this process by sharing your list of medications with any doctor who is caring for you, even if they were prescribed by a different doctor.

> There are health-care benefits
> in having your pharmacist
> as a member of your team and
> filling all your prescriptions
> at one pharmacy.

How Private Drug Plans Work

The majority of people with private medical insurance have a drug benefit as part of their policies. From an expense perspective, it is the fastest-growing component of health insurance, and has been for many years. As the cost of drug benefit plans have risen, insurance companies have been working to manage the increase through tighter constraints and regulations.

Insurance companies base their prescription plans on what is called a **drug formulary,** which is the list of drugs that the insurance plan prefers your doctors to dispense. The formulary is selected by a Pharmacy and Therapeutics Committee, which is made up of physicians and pharmacists. The function of the committee is to track medical practice and pharmaceutical developments and decide if and how the insurance company will insure a drug. Be aware that the insurance drug plans do not cover all classes of drugs. For instance, there is a category called lifestyle drugs, which many insurance companies do not cover. Examples in this class include diet pills and male potency drugs. Insurance companies also may not cover all medicines within a class. For instance, they may not include all anti-depressants in their formulary.

How drugs are priced and how much an insurance company is willing to pay has a lot to do with how long a drug has been available. Drugs are most expensive when they first enter the market because the company that developed it has an exclusive right to it while it is under a patent. This is when the drug goes by a **brand name** only. With no competition, the price of the drug is usually quite high.

Once the patent expires, other pharmaceutical companies can make the drug, which is then sold under its **chemical or generic name.** The generic drug is significantly cheaper than the brand name. Once generic drugs hit the market, insurance companies want doctors to prescribe them as a cost-saving measure.

• How does a drug get on the formulary?

When a new drug is first released, it most likely will not be on the drug company formulary. The insurance company's Pharmacy and Therapeutics Committee won't evaluate a new drug until there is patient demand, physician input, or they do their own research. The Pharmacy and Therapeutics Committee can then elect to add the drug to their formulary. When the patent on the medicine expires, the committee will usually add the generic form to the formulary and eliminate the brand name.

For many medical conditions, there are multiple drugs that can be used. Sometimes, the committee wants to limit the choices a patient has. This is often because the insurance company can pay less for one drug than another. If the committee feels a certain class of drugs is equally effective, it may select only one or a few for the formulary, based on the lowest price. This is particularly true if the health insurance plan is more heavily managed.

- **How do generic drugs differ from brand-name drugs?**
  Generics drugs, by law, are required to contain the identical active (healing) ingredient as the brand-name drugs. However, they are not required to contain the same inactive ingredients— the other substances used to form a capsule or pill. Supporters of this regulation feel that only the active ingredients are important to the patient. For the most part, this seems to be quite true. I routinely use generic medications. On occasion, however, someone will get an adverse effect from an inactive ingredient in a drug. If this happens, you should not have a problem getting the insurance company to accept the brand name, though you will still pay more for it.

Therapeutics Are Not Generics

Do not confuse generic substitutions and **therapeutic substitutions**. They are not the same. Unlike generics, therapeutic substitutions do not contain the same active ingredients found in the brand-name drugs. The intent of a therapeutic substitution is to replace a drug with a different drug that will have the same healing effect. **The active ingredients are different.**

Sometimes an insurance company will take a drug off its formulary and replace it with a different drug from the same therapeutic class. They either select an already-lower-cost drug or contract to buy a large quantity of a given drug from a drug manufacturer at a reduced rate. They then want all the patients in their plan who are taking drugs in the same class to use the one they purchased in bulk.

For example, people frequently talk about taking statins (cholesterol-lowering drugs). An insurance company may contract to buy a large supply of one statin and then want to move all the patients taking other statins to this one drug. **This means the active ingredient the patient is taking will change, and it is possible that he won't respond the same to the new drug.**

Therapeutic substitutions may work for many or most patients, but I don't believe they work for all. If your medication is changed as part of a therapeutic substitution and you do not respond well to the new drug or you have bothersome side effects from it, talk to your doctor. **Your doctor can usually file an appeal with the insurance company to prescribe your original drug.**

> Therapeutic substitutions are not the same as generic substitutions. Talk to your doctor if a therapeutic substitution is recommended.

- **How do I get my drugs added to the formulary?**

  The best drug plan for you is one that includes the prescription medications that you take. Can you do anything about that? I believe the answer to this question is "yes." I think the best strategy is to get your physician to contact your insurance company's Pharmacy and Therapeutics Committee and request inclusion of the drugs you need in the formulary. This is one of those times when **your doctor can be a much more powerful voice for you than if you called personally.** Better still, if you have more than one doctor providing your care (a family practitioner and a cardiologist, for instance), get them both to contact your insurance company. I know from personal experience as a medical insurance executive that drugs more often get added to the insurance formularies when physicians make a case for needing access to them. Get your partner in health care to go to bat for you.

> You need to understand your insurance drug plan and the difference between generic drugs, brand-name drugs, and nonformulary drugs.

Medicare Is Even More Complicated

If you have been on Medicare without a supplement policy, you were not entitled to a drug reimbursement until January 1, 2006.

This is when **Medicare Part D** went into effect—launched, unfortunately, with a lot of confusion over myriad choices with a variety of exceptions. I will leave it at that. Here is the essence of what Part D is all about.

Although it is a government program, it is provided through a variety of private insurance companies. This means that if you want to sign up for Medicare Part D, you have to select from a variety of private insurance plans that provide this service to eligible Medicare participant. Participation is voluntary.

You have to pay a monthly premium to the insurance company for the benefit. If you don't sign up during the first open-enrollment period for which you are eligible, the penalty is a higher premium. The medications offered will vary from plan to plan, and the number of drugs available in these formularies are limited for most plans. You want to pick the plan that requires you to make the fewest changes in the medications you take. If changes are required, work with your doctor to select the new drug that is best for you.

Not all pharmacies are included in all plans. If you like to use a specific pharmacy, you want to select a plan that has your pharmacy in its network.

To say Medicare D is complex and difficult to understand is an understatement, but there are some good Web sites that can help you learn more about this plan. They include **www.medicare.gov** and **www.aarp.org**. There may be other sites with information that you know you can trust; just be careful when searching the Web to make sure that you are getting accurate information. (See chapter 17 for guidelines on using the Internet.) You can also call the Medicare offices directly at **1-800-MEDICARE**.

Be aware that **if you use several expensive prescriptions, the out-of-pocket cost to the Medicare Part D participant for the medications can still be significant,** even with the newest pharmacy benefit. This is how it works:

- There is an initial annual $250 deductible (the amount you have to pay before the plan pays you any benefit).
- There is a 25 percent co-pay on the next $2,000 (after you have met your deductible).

- You pay the next $2,850 yourself. This is called the coverage gap, or the doughnut hole. By this point, you have paid $3,600 out-of-pocket for a total of $5,100 worth of drugs (having received $1,500 in drug benefits).
- Medicare will then begin paying again under its catastrophic drug benefit. This coverage is quite good and amounts to about 95 percent of the cost of your prescription drugs from then until the end of the insurance year.
- On each January 1, the payment schedule starts all over again.

Medicare Part D is in its infancy, and the program likely will change over time.

> A new Medicare pharmacy benefit
> program began in 2006. You want
> to fully understand it.

• What does it mean to me if I have Original Medicare with a Medigap policy?

If you are already enrolled in Medicare and have a Medigap policy with a drug benefit, then you can opt to continue that policy and forgo Medicare Part D. This is an individual decision, and you need to carefully evaluate formularies and the expenses of both plans to decide which is best for you.

As of January 1, 2006, new enrollees are no longer allowed to sign up for a drug benefit through Medigap. Drug plans are now offered to new retirees only through Medicare Part D.

• What if I have a Medicare Advantage Plan?

Most Medicare Advantage plans have a drug benefit. You need to study the details of your plan to make a wise decision. I know how hard it often is to understand insurance plans. However, the wise medical advocate can best get the coverage he wants by putting in the effort. To find out more about Medicare Advantage plans, see page 215.

• How does this apply if I am a retiree with a health insurance benefit from my former employer?

Some retirees still receive their health care coverage through an employer-sponsored retirement health plan. If you are in this group, you know that this policy is integrated into your Medicare benefit. Depending on the nature of the plan you are in, the drug benefit will vary. If you have any questions, often a good place to start is the human resources department at your former employer.

Smart and Safe Strategies

• **What do I do if I am going on vacation and will run out of a medicine?**

If you are going away on vacation, make sure you have enough medication to see you through. Pharmacies often will not refill a prescription in advance without a notice from your doctor. Your insurance company will also have controls in place to limit how often you can refill a prescription.

This is another example why your pharmacist should be a member of your medical team. Review all your prescriptions and bring those that will run out to your pharmacist. Tell him your vacation dates and ask him to file a request with the insurance company for early refills to carry you through your vacation. If your pharmacist has concerns about any of the medications, ask him to check with your doctor first. In my experience as a physician and an insurance executive, I have seen this strategy work well to avoid a medication shortage during vacations.

• **Are there other ways to save money on my medicines?**

Many insurance companies will allow you to get a 3-month supply of medication for chronic conditions. They often charge less for a single 3-month refill, usually about two-thirds of what you would pay if you filled the prescription once a month for 3 months. (Essentially, it's like buy two, get one free, if you buy it all at once.)

Another strategy is to use a mail-in pharmacy option if your insurance company has one. This option allows patients to order prescriptions by mail at a lower co-pay than if they go to a pharmacy. It's more convenient to have your prescriptions delivered to your mailbox, but it does mean you have to keep track of and plan for your refills. You have to order them leaving enough lead time for processing and shipping, usually 10 to 14 days. **When you use the mail-order pharmacy for a standard 90-day supply of your long-term medications, you are optimizing your pharmacy benefit.**

The Risks in Taking Drugs

As I already mentioned, drugs that in and of themselves are safe can be dangerous when one or a few are mixed. Always make sure that your doctors and your primary-care physician, in particular, are up-to-date on the drugs you are taking. If your doctor changes a drug, take notice if you experience any side effects. If so, let your doctor know immediately. This is especially true if you are taking a therapeutic substitute. It also applies if you are taking a drug for the first time.

> FOR INSTANCE...
> Risa is a registered nurse who was put on a new medication. She began having progressive weakness and dizziness, and one day blacked out for a few moments. She was concerned and told me that if it happened again, she was going to call her doctor. I told her to stop taking the drug and call her doctor immediately. It turned out that another dose could have precipitated an even more serious, even potentially fatal, reaction.

Now this is a very bright, well-trained nurse. If she didn't realize that she was experiencing side-effects from a new drug, think how much harder it is for the average patient.

The key thing to remember is that you have to **respect the risks as well as the benefits of medications and listen to your body**.

My final word of advice on medication is to always make sure that you double-check your prescriptions. Pharmacists work hard to prevent mistakes, but with millions of prescriptions being filled each day, errors do happen. When you pick up your prescription:

- Read the label to make sure the prescription is for you.
- Look carefully to see that the label reflects the drug name and strength your doctor told you to expect.
- Open the bottle, and if you have had the medicine before, check to make sure it is the same medicine as before.
- If the label has an error, or the pills look different than before, ask the pharmacist about it.
- If you are obtaining a refill of a generic drug, the pharmacy may have changed suppliers. Don't assume this—ask the pharmacist!

> Double-check your prescriptions before you leave the pharmacy!

Key Take Home Messages

- Your drug benefit is one of the most important parts of your health insurance.

- You need to understand your insurance drug plan and the difference between brand-name drugs, generic drugs, and therapeutic substitutions.

- If you are on Medicare, make sure you understand the drug plan options before you choose one.

- Before you go on vacation, make sure you have enough medications.

- Using one pharmacy provides a complete electronic record of your medications and alerts your pharmacist to possible dangerous drug interactions.

- Respect the risks as well as the benefits of medications.

- Double-check your prescription before you leave the pharmacy.

23

THE INSURANCE COMPANY IS NOT THE BOSS!

How should I respond to a denial?

How can a case manager help me?

What do I do if my case manager says "no"?

If the Insurance Company Says "No!"

You have a contract with your insurance company that in essence says that you will pay premiums, and the insurance will pay for your medical care. As your own medical advocate you want to control:

- What care you receive.
- When you receive it.
- Who you receive it from.

Insurance companies also wants to control these same three things, but their sole interest is in limiting what they are going to cost. They do this through your benefit contract that defines:

- What care you insurance will cover.
- Who your insurance wants to pay to provide it.

The most common source of conflict with a medical insurance company is a denied referral for a patient to see another doctor. If you need medical care that your insurance company says it will not cover, there are strategies you can employ to get your insurance company to see things your way. I can tell you from my combined experience as a physician, a medical insurance executive, and a patient: **You don't have to take "no" for an answer!**

- ## How should I respond to a denial?
  In order to plan your response you first need to understand why the insurance company is saying "no." This can happen because:

- You are requesting a non-covered benefit.
- You want to see an out-of-network doctor or go to an out-of-network facility.

In both instances your policy offers a variety of covered options and **the insurance company wants you to use one of them.** The denial is the insurance company's way of pushing you to use a covered option. You don't have to. As your own medical advocate there are important tactics you can use to get your own way. First, arm yourself with this information:

- Get your doctor's insight as to why your request was denied and get her to be your ally.
- Know how your physician network works so you can cogently relate why it is not adequate for you in your particular circumstance.
- Request that you be assigned to an insurance company case manager and know how to effectively work with one.
- Know when it is better to have your doctor talk to directly to the insurance company's medical director on your behalf.
- Understand and be ready to use the Appeals Process.
- Don't let the insurance company create any unnecessary delays in your care.

> There are strategies you can use to get your insurance company to see things your way.

Your Doctor Is Your Ally

Doctor's deal with insurance companies all the time. Your doctor can frequently tell you why your referral was denied, so **talk to your doctor before you call your insurance company.** It is possible your doctor may not have supported the request, even though she allowed it. If this is the case, then it is really not an insurance issue, but a medical care issue. It's always possible that your doctor made the referral knowing it will be turned down but did so in order to avoid having a conflict with you. This shifts the blame from the doctor to the insurance company.

If you discover that your doctor does not believe the referral was medically indicated, then you need to talk with your doctor and smooth out your communication. You want your doctor to be able to tell you no when she feels something is not in your medical best interest even if you ask for it.

It is not unusual for your insurance company to deny a referral to see a doctor that is out of the network. Again, your doctor-partner is your ally. If you had specifically chosen the referral doctor, discuss the choice with your doctor. Possibly she can guide you to someone within your network you are not aware of who is an equal or even a better option than your first choice. If not, work with your doctor to define why your choice is medically a better choice. For instance, what special skills does your choice possess that you cannot get from any of the in-network doctors? **You have already paid for your insurance; you sure don't want to pay twice!**

The Role of a Case Manager

Insurance companies employ **case managers to help coordinate the care of individual clients who have complex medical problems.** All case managers are nurses and their job is to help you in a way that is most efficient—that is, the least expensive.

- **How can a case manager help me?**
  It is very important to establish a good relationship with your case manager because she is the one who can help you obtain an exception to the usual rules of the insurance company. In making your case, **keep in mind the key rule of the insurance company: The best medical care is the cheapest medical care.**

  For example, you may be able to state that what you want may cost more in the short run, but it will save money in the long term. Be prepared to make a case that it is a benefit to the insurance company as well as yourself. If you want the insurance company to pay for a benefit that is not covered, it is possible to get it if you can show that it will avoid the need for more costly covered benefits. A case manager may be able to exchange benefits for you. These are the type of tactics you need to use on your case manager. Your doctor can help you prepare your argument. **You need to present it as a win-win strategy—it is good for you as well as the insurance company.**

> Invite your case manager to be part of your health care team.

If you have a chronic or complex illness I believe it is essential for you to request the assistance of a case manager. Many delays can be encountered with an illness that requires seeing multiple doctors and getting a large number of tests or treatments. Case managers can help coordinate appointments, processes, and getting test results in a timely manner.

- **What do I do if my case manager says "no"?**
  If you are not getting success through your case manager, don't give up. **Go back to your doctor and get her to go to bat for you.** If the case manager is not budging, ask your doctor to call the insurance company's **Medical Director.** It is amazing how often a call from a doctor can break an impasse between a patient and her insurance company. Doctor to doctor conversations are often the most effective way to get your message across.

> If you can't get the case manager to solve your problem, get your doctor to call the insurance company Medical Director.

The Appeal Process—Use It!

Just like a verdict can be appealed in a court of law, an insurance company decision can be appealed. Every insurance company has an appeals process. Unlike the legal system, you don't have to wait months or even years for your case to be heard. Generally, this is what happens.

If your efforts with a case manager and the Medical Director fail, your next step can be to appeal the decision. There are several avenues of appeal:

- **The insurance company appeal process.** Every insurance company has a formal appeals process. If you end up going this route, follow the guidelines of the process carefully.

You don't want needless delays while the insurance company tells you that you didn't follow the rules.

- **Go to the CEO.** If you still can not make progress, write to the CEO of the insurance company. Many companies are very sensitive about consumers who write directly to the CEO. This strategy can often get your request reviewed by people who are more concerned about consumer good will.
- **Go to your state Insurance Commissioner.** Every state has an insurance commissioner who is responsible for regulating the insurance companies in that state. If you cannot get satisfaction from your insurance company, you can make an appeal to the insurance commissioner. You can find out about how your state's process works by contacting **www.naic.org**.

Time Is Critical

Time is often critical when it comes to health care, so make sure to state clearly the urgency of your need with whomever you are dealing. Using patience with a process is often a good strategy, but if the medical issue is urgent, **don't accept delays.**

> You have many options if your health plan says "no." Use them all if necessary!

If you are working with a case manager or appealing a decision, discuss the timeline and hold people to it. You don't want to prolong your medical problem! If you need to repeatedly make calls or even go to their offices, do so. It is up to you to highlight the urgency of your care. **Being assertive does pay off.**

FOR EXAMPLE...
A man I know was being cared for at an outstanding teaching hospital for a brain tumor that, unfortunately, was very close to vital structures. His neurosurgeon, who was a

professor at the medical school, said he could not safely remove it without risking major post-operative paralysis. However, there was a new, safer technique being used at another university hospital some distance away. The patient worked with his doctor to get a referral to have the surgery done at the other center, which was out-of-network. He got the referral but his insurance company wouldn't approve it. My friend worked on his insurance company. He sent literature on the new procedure; he got his doctor to write a letter of support; he communicated with his case manager. Finally, his persistence paid off, and the insurance company approved the surgery. He had the procedure and came through it miraculously.

This is more than a wonderful story. It is an example of how **you can impact the quality of your care if you persist in your efforts to get the care you believe you need. In the end, getting what you need to protect your health is what matters the most.** By using the knowledge and skills you learned in this book **you can get:**

- **The medical care you want.**
- **When you want it.**
- **From whom you want it.**

You can do this in your doctor's office, in the hospital, and with your insurance company. You now have the skills. **Don't take no for an answer!**

Key Take Home Messages

- Get your doctor to go to bat for you.
- Request the assistance of a case manager.
- Take advantage of the appeal processes.
- Establish a timeline and don't accept delays.
- Never accept "no" for an answer.

INDEX

About the Author

Bob Sheff, M.D., received his medical training as a radiologist at U.C.L.A. and Johns Hopkins Medical Center. His expertise in medical insurance comes from his long career as an administrator for one of the largest medical managed-care systems in the United States. He became The Medical Mentor by helping friends and family who were faced with sickness and hospitalization to navigate the complicated medical health system; the word spread, and he began working with other patients in his community and beyond. Now semi-retired, Dr. Sheff continues to devote his time to helping people address their medical concerns, and in *The Medical Mentor* he encourages readers to learn to take charge of their own health. He lives in Columbia, Maryland.
Visit his website at **www.themedicalmentor.net**.